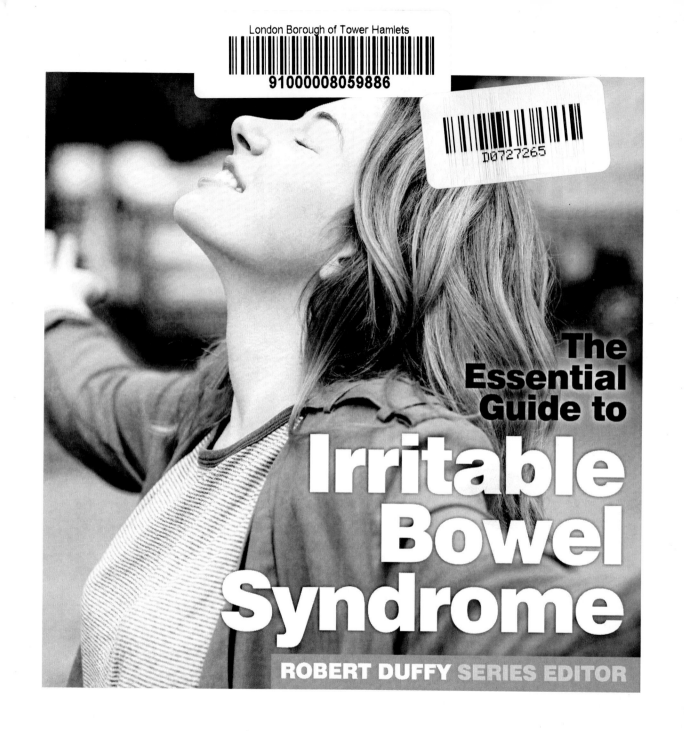

The Essential Guide to

Irritable Bowel Syndrome

ROBERT DUFFY SERIES EDITOR

Published in Great Britain in 2018 by

need2know

Remus House
Coltsfoot Drive
Peterborough
PE2 9BF
Telephone 01733 898103
www.need2knowbooks.co.uk

Contents

Chapter 13: Conclusion 99

Chapter 14: Frequently Asked Questions 103

Chapter 15: Case Studies 107

Help List 111

Introduction

Ask around any dinner table or bar and you can be almost certain that there will be someone there who suffers with Irritable Bowel Syndrome (IBS). Abdominal pain, constipation, frequent bowel motions, bloating, headaches and depression are just some of the symptoms they're probably dealing with on a regular basis.

Research suggests that as many as eight million people in the UK have IBS. While it's fair to say that most of us suffer with diarrhoea, constipation, wind, a bloated stomach or abdominal pain at some point in our lives, how do you know if you've got IBS?

IBS is an umbrella term used to explain a whole range of symptoms which are unrelated to a specific medical condition. It's described as a functional disorder because the way that the bowel normally operates or 'functions' is affected.

Research has provided a number of explanations as to why we're experiencing it. Some experts believe IBS is linked to stress, and the National Health Service (NHS) reports up to 60% of people with IBS experience psychological symptoms like anxiety, nervous headaches and depression.

Symptoms appear to be triggered by many different factors and stress is by no means believed to be the only cause. Food intolerances, gender, age and lifestyle factors are also involved. But whatever the cause and wherever it came from, one in 10 people suffer severely enough to seek advice from their GP.

Whether you think you've got it, or know someone who has, this book will give you the lowdown on IBS. If you've already been diagnosed, you might be feeling frustrated by the lack of understanding and advice available, or even the suggestion that your condition isn't 'real'. This book aims to bring together the necessary information needed for you to take control and gain more understanding of the condition. If modern-day stress really is a major contributor, how do you recognise that how you're feeling is affecting your digestion and make the appropriate changes for good digestive health?

IBS affects everyone differently. This book outlines the many different ways to treat symptoms and explores positive ways to accept, reduce and even reverse IBS: from conventional or alternative medicine to diet and stress management – no stone is left unturned.

You'll also get advice on the emotional aspects of IBS and the effects it can have on your relationships and everyday life. There's information on red flag symptoms, the role of the digestive system, diagnosis, prevention and the close relationship between the bowels and the brain.

As IBS tends to be more prevalent in women, there's a chapter dedicated to them to help them deal with IBS during their periods when hormones and premenstrual tension can upset the bowels and exacerbate symptoms. Equally, because IBS is often cited as being a disease which starts early on in life (for many people in their teens) this book aims to explain IBS in simple terms so that younger readers aren't overwhelmed by complicated medical terms.

At the end you'll find a FAQ (frequently asked questions) section dispelling some of the common myths about IBS, along with some real life case studies and a list of useful organisations.

I was introduced to the principles of an Austrian physician, Dr F. X. Mayr, on a press trip to the Viva Mayr health resort in Austria, and would especially like to thank Dr Harald and Dr Christine Stossier at the Viva Mayr for their top class treatment and advice. Their knowledge has inspired several parts of this book and has transformed my own eating habits. You'll learn more about the Mayr approach to IBS and digestion in the later chapters.

Since IBS symptoms are very treatable, this book aims to help you find simple solutions, taking into account lifestyle, occupation and personality type. Ultimately, the best cure for IBS is to understand it and know what triggers it for you, as well as how to avoid the frequency and intensity of the symptoms.

Acknowledgements

While researching and writing this book I interviewed several experts in the area of digestion and treatment of IBS, and would like to thank them for their invaluable contribution:

Susie Perry, a nutritional therapist, writer and founder of the Nurturing Spirit nutritional therapy practice based in East Sussex, for her clinical expertise and experience in treating patients with IBS and other digestive disorders.

Dr Suneil Kapadia, consultant gastroenterologist at New Cross Hospital, Royal Wolverhampton NHS Trust, for his contribution in chapter 6 about diagnosing and treating IBS.

Dr Harald Stossier, physician, Mayr practitioner and medical director of the Viva Centre, Viva Mayr, Austria, for his invaluable input regarding the Mayr approach to healthy digestion and optimum health.

Andrew Spence, Dip PDMSM, MNCH (Acc) of the Spence Practice, East Sussex, a solution-focused hypnotherapist and life coach, for his clinical experience and expertise on treating IBS using hypnotherapy and mind-over-matter techniques.

Disclaimer

This book is for general information on Irritable Bowel Syndrome only. It is not intended to replace professional medical advice. The book can be used alongside medical advice but readers are strongly advised to see their GP rather than using the book as a diagnosis or cure for IBS.

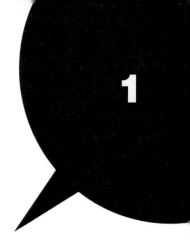
What Is Irritable Bowel Syndrome?

I rritable Bowel Syndrome (IBS) is a chronic bowel disorder that is thought to affect around eight million people in the UK today. IBS is used as an umbrella term to describe the list of symptoms which relate to a disturbance in the bowel's function, rather than a structural abnormality or underlying illness which would explain the symptoms. Essentially, this means that the function of the gut is upset but all other parts look perfectly normal.

IBS is also sometimes referred to as spastic colon or spastic constipation.

It's a mystery

IBS is often described as a baffling and mysterious disease because no two people are affected in the same way, and because no one really knows where it came from or exactly what causes it. Mystery aside, statistics suggest that one third of the UK's population experience IBS symptoms at some point in their lives, making the condition very real.

Some people experience mild symptoms and others feel debilitated and distressed by it. Let's face it, talking about how often you go to the toilet and the state of your stools is not a subject many of us are comfortable with, especially if and when you dare to do so you're deemed a hypochondriac with a simple bout of diarrhoea!

Without the right kind of advice or support, you may start to think there is little hope of ever feeling well again.

Why have I got it?

If you have IBS, you probably feel that you need to open your bowels urgently and that your stools vary in consistency: sometimes hard but at other times loose and watery. One day you might have constipation, another day diarrhoea.

IBS can seem to strike from nowhere and it can be confusing to understand why and how to treat it, especially as the symptoms can change. New ones can appear without warning and methods for managing the condition can seem to suddenly stop working.

It's difficult to pinpoint the exact cause of IBS but as it's a 'functional' disorder, it means that certain things are causing the digestive system to behave the way that it does. Since IBS is a modern disease, many health experts believe it has arisen as a result of stress and our fast-paced lifestyles.

Stress can affect the functioning of an ordinarily healthy digestive system, but there are several other causes to consider. Some experts believe IBS could be linked to a person's genetic make-up or family history. Other causes include diet and a person's general attitude to life. It's also believed that people with IBS have more sensitivity in their gut so they react to stress more easily than those with less sensitive guts. Their IBS could initially have been triggered by an upsetting emotional event.

One thing for certain is that IBS affects a person's quality of life and, unlike other illnesses, it doesn't tend to go away after two weeks of prescribed medication.

Possible causes of IBS

- Imbalances in the gut's flora (the natural or 'friendly' bacteria).

- A bacterial infection or parasitic infection, after which IBS symptoms begin.

- Allergies and intolerance to products like fructose, lactose, gluten or wheat.

- Stress.

- Eating too quickly and not digesting food properly (especially when anxious).

- Eating a diet rich in sugar, alcohol, fatty and processed foods and not eating enough fibre (or even the wrong type of fibre – more about this in chapter 8).

IBS symptoms can mimic other digestive disorders, so it's not always clear when someone actually has IBS. There are some 'red flag' symptoms you should be aware of.

If you recognise any of the causes above and any of the symptoms listed below, it is strongly recommended that you book an appointment to see your GP to rule out other serious conditions such as colon cancer and inflammatory bowel disease.

Red flag symptoms

- Bleeding from the rectum.

- Blood with the stools.

- Indigestion-type pain that keeps you awake at night.

- Weight loss.

- Anaemia.

- Being aged over 45 and having a family history of cancer or inflammatory bowel disease.

'IBS symptoms can mimic other digestive disorders, so it's not always clear when someone actually has IBS.'

What you eat

Diet plays a large part in how well your gut is working, but did you know that eating too fast and not chewing your food properly can seriously aggravate the condition? You can learn more about the importance of chewing and eating a healthy diet in chapters 8, 9 and 10.

Don't worry

If you're diagnosed with IBS, the condition is likely to persist for some time. However, symptoms can come and go and for long periods of time they may even disappear completely. Reassuringly, IBS isn't life threatening – it doesn't necessarily lead to more serious conditions and the symptoms can be treated and managed.

In the following chapters you'll discover solutions to benefit you, taking into account your lifestyle, occupation and personality. Ultimately, the best cure for IBS is to understand what triggers it and to learn how to avoid the frequency and intensity of the symptoms.

Action points

- Buy a new notebook to keep a 'trigger diary' (see template on page 14). The purpose of the diary is to help you take note of what you eat for breakfast, lunch and dinner every day. You can even include all the snacks you had in between (yes, including that bar of chocolate or handful of peanuts!). Make sure you also include sauces, dips or marinades.

- Also include alcohol and where you ate your food, i.e. relaxed at home, on the go, standing up or at your desk or workplace. This is a free and simple way to highlight any troublesome foods and drinks, as well as behavioural contributors (for example, you may find you have abdominal pain or need to rush to the toilet after eating in a hurry or when you're upset).

- As well as listing food, you can also begin grading each day's symptoms on a scale of 0 to 10 (with 10 being bad and 0 being non-existent) according to how bad they were. Keeping a record of when symptoms occur can be useful because if certain foods or events (such as interactions with a difficult colleague at work, an argument with your parents, problems on public transport or being late for an important event) can be identified as triggers, you can learn how to deal with the stress of these and in turn reduce the IBS symptoms.

- Write details such as whether it was a good and productive day, whether you got to socialise with friends or family, found time to relax with a magazine, music or book or do some exercise. Maybe you felt excited, sad, anxious, stressed or nervous. Try to be honest about your mood and feelings on each day so that you can begin to see if there is a connection between how you feel and how well your bowels function.

- Complete the IBS diary for a period of 14 days, after which time you may begin to notice patterns forming. More focused tests can then be applied by eliminating suspected trigger items from the diet for a subsequent 14-day period.

This is just the beginning of understanding your IBS. There will be more about diet and nutrition in chapter 9 with advice and recommendations from a nutritional therapist and digestive experts.

Trigger diary template

Fill in the following table over the next two weeks, including weekends.

Meals	Day 1	Day 2	Day 3	Day 4	Day 5	Day 6	Day 7
Breakfast							
Lunch							
Dinner							
Snacks							
Drinks							
Comments							
Mood							

Comments note what symptoms you had and how bad they were on a scale of 0-10, with 0 being none and 10 being severe.

Mood on a scale of 0-10, with 0 being low and 10 being fantastic, note your mood on that particular day.

Summing Up

Now you know you're not alone. There are literally millions of other people who may be experiencing very similar symptoms to you at this very moment. One of the key points to remember is that although IBS is a mysterious disease, it's certainly not a life-threatening one. Now that you've got a basic understanding of the condition and how to define it, hopefully some of the confusion or uncertainty will be lifted and you will be able to get your head around whether you (or someone close to you) actually have IBS. Following the action points on page 12 will help you gain more understanding of your IBS and when and how it occurs.

Well done! You're now on the path to taking control of your IBS rather than allowing it to control you.

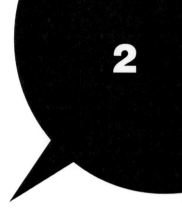

2

Understanding Your Digestive System

t's easy to forget that our bodies are complex machines and that our whole system needs to be working in harmony to enjoy optimum health.

Digestion is the process by which food and drink is broken down into small parts that the body can use to build cells and give you energy.

Here are some useful terms:

- Ingestion = taking food into the mouth.
- Mastication = chewing food and the salivary action.
- Deglutition = swallowing.

The digestive process takes place in a long coiled tube (around 27 feet in size) that extends from the mouth to the anus called the alimentary canal or the gut. The alimentary canal is responsible for ingestion, digestion, absorption and egestion (elimination or, put simply, going to the toilet).

Food is broken down by the teeth (the chewing action) and muscles in the alimentary canal which squeeze food and push it from one end to the other in a process known as peristalsis. As the food moves down the alimentary canal, digestive juices soften and lubricate it and digestive enzymes break the food down chemically.

The digestive organs process food and fluids so that nutrients can be absorbed from the intestines and circulated around the body. When digested food arrives in the large intestine, most of the nutrient content has been absorbed. Food residues which haven't been digested become faeces. Water is absorbed from the undigested food that enters the colon to make the faeces which are then removed from the body when you go to the toilet.

'The digestive system physically and chemically breaks down food to get rid of what the body doesn't need.'

How long does the body take to digest food?

In a healthy person the process of digestion (the time from when the food enters your mouth to elimination) takes between 12 and 24 hours. Two to three bowel movements each day, i.e. going to the toilet after each meal, is considered to be healthy (though not necessarily the case for us all!).Infrequent bowel movements can allow toxins from undigested food to stay in the colon and affect your overall health and energy.

The organs of the digestive system

There are many different parts to the digestive system: the oral cavity, throat, oesophagus (a muscular tube), stomach and the small and large intestines. There are also the salivary glands in the mouth, the liver, gall bladder, the pancreas and the many mucous glands in the stomach and intestines, with the stomach being the widest part of the digestive tract.

What is peristalsis and how does it work?

Peristalsis is a series of smooth-muscle contractions which move the contents of the bowels along. When food is swallowed, it passes down to the stomach and becomes a fluid. This then passes through to the small intestine where most of the nutrients are absorbed. The remaining waste products are collected in the colon and rectum and are emptied during a bowel movement.

You'll be completely unaware of peristalsis when it's working properly, but when peristalsis is irregular you're likely to feel discomfort or pain. You might experience diarrhoea and/or constipation, bloating and flatulence – all very typical IBS symptoms.

IBS is a loss of co-ordination of these muscular contractions.

The importance of the colon

The colon is responsible for transferring waste material from the small intestine to the rectum, and healthy functioning of the colon is vital. The colon converts food (known as 'chyme') into faeces for excretion, absorbing water from chyme and changing it from liquid into solid which is then released from the body. Inside the colon are lots of different varieties of bacteria (flora) which help digestion and maintain good health.

The importance of chewing

It's a common belief that digestion begins when food gets to the stomach and many people think that digestion merely means eating some food then going to the toilet and producing a stool. But proper digestion involves much more and there are many mechanical and chemical processes which must take place in order for food to be broken down.

Chewing food properly helps begin the digestive process – enzymes in your saliva begin to break down food. If the food isn't chewed properly, it's harder for your body to digest and absorb nutrients.

The action of chewing breaks down food molecules into smaller particles which, apart from making food smaller and easier to swallow, aids digestion. The saliva in the mouth helps to lubricate the food, again making it easier to swallow, but the enzymes in the saliva also help break down the food.

'Although digestion begins in the mouth, you could say that it truly begins as soon as you see or smell food, when the saliva is activated!'

Eating slowly and calmly

Most of us rush through our days, racing through our activities to get everything done. When it comes to eating, we gobble food down and hurry on to the next thing in our chaotic lives. The sad fact is that this rushing and racing means we don't get to enjoy each precious moment and, to coin the old adage, stop and smell the roses.

This also applies to our eating habits. How common it is today for office workers to grab a sandwich at their desk while checking emails or continuing to write a report, barely even noticing what they're eating, the flavour or texture. The same goes for teenagers who eat on the hoof, buying takeaway food in their lunch hour then eating it on their walk back to school.

For good health, and fundamentally for good digestive health, it's extremely important to eat slowly and to make time to sit down and eat in a relaxed, unhurried manner. Doing so could help avoid wind, bloating, uncomfortable indigestion and many IBS symptoms. There'll be more about this in later chapters which look in more detail at the effects of stress on the digestive system.

'What you eat is obviously of great importance but when and how you eat it is of equal importance.'

Dr Harald Stossier, medical director, the Viva Mayr Health Resort, Austria.

Summing Up

That's the digestive system in a nutshell. We know that a strong digestive system will help us to enjoy good health and longevity. When the digestive system works efficiently, it can absorb the vitamins and minerals we need to be healthy. If we don't pay attention to what, how and when we eat, our digestive systems will suffer.

It may seem impossible at this stage to imagine how you're going to suddenly start slowing down to make more time for relaxed eating but there will be plenty of tips and advice in the later chapters. Awareness is the first stage for positive change.

3

Who Gets IBS?

IBS can affect anyone and everyone. None of us have perfectly functioning bowels all of the time and according to the Gut Trust, between 10% and 20% of people living in Western countries fulfil the diagnostic criteria for IBS at any given time.

Plenty of data suggests that women are more susceptible to IBS than men (the NHS report that IBS is twice as common in women, particularly bloating and wind) and although it tends to be most common in people between the ages of 20 and 40, IBS can also affect babies and elderly people. It is also widely seen as a modern and 'Western' condition.

Some people can have attacks which last days or weeks, while other people have recurrent attacks during their lives. This chapter explores who gets IBS, why and when, and whether you can actually prevent it.

Women vs. men

IBS Research Appeal is a registered UK charity based at Central Middlesex Hospital in London which funds a research programme into the causes and treatments of IBS. It is directed by a leading gastroenterologist, Professor David Silk, MD, FRCP. The charity claims that women are three times more likely to be seen in their specialist clinic and at other clinics the hospital has been in contact with during their research than men.

Is this because women are more likely to go and talk about their bodily symptoms? Could men be suffering in silence, believing that their symptoms don't warrant the doctor's time? This could indeed be the case; the charity also carried out a symptom questionnaire survey and received responses from only half the amount of men compared to women. So whether men simply didn't have the time or inclination to fill out the questionnaire or they really don't suffer as much as women is open to interpretation!

However, experts believe women may be more susceptible to IBS than men because emotional and psychological issues like depression and anxiety (which can trigger IBS symptoms and, indeed, vice versa) are twice as common in women as they are in men. IBS could also be more common in women because their menstrual cycle makes symptoms such as abdominal pain or constipation worse. There is more about this in chapter 7.

'I constantly feel like I've got a balloon strapped to my front which I want someone to burst with a pin.'

Alan, IBS sufferer, aged 40, Brighton.

When does IBS first strike?

The NHS says that IBS is one of the most common gastrointestinal conditions in the UK and that it normally develops in people aged between 20 and 30.

Men tend to suffer with IBS from a younger age and mainly experience diarrhoea, while women tend to get it in their 20s or 30s and more commonly experience constipation. But, ultimately, IBS can affect anyone at any age, even infants.

Children

According to the Gut Trust, indigestion can start at infancy. Babies can experience colic in the first few months of life which can be brought on by intestinal spasm, over-feeding or stress about being left alone. This pain can cause them to refuse feeds.

Small children can also experience diarrhoea even when there are no other symptoms. Constipation is quite common, usually in boys more than girls. According to figures from the Gut Trust, recurrent abdominal pain syndrome occurs in about 25% of children between the ages of five and 12.

Teenagers

The teenage years can be an angst-ridden and difficult time. Peer pressure, exams, spots, changing bodies, deepening voices and unfamiliar emotions are all factors which could add to stress and trigger IBS. Adolescence is particularly tough, and teenagers suffering with IBS may be embarrassed and unwilling to talk to anyone about it, thus feeling quite isolated (see chapter 12 for help and advice on this).

When is IBS most likely to strike?

The NHS says that, on average, symptoms start around the age of 15 but diagnosis is most likely to occur between the ages of 30 and 40. Doctors believe that people over the age of 40 have an increased chance that their IBS-compatible symptoms could be due to other more serious diseases of the bowel (such as bowel cancer) and more active investigation should be carried out. (Of course, it's quite likely that their symptoms are just IBS-related, but anyone over 40 is considered to be at higher risk so this needs to be taken into account.)

Why is IBS only a Western condition?

People in developing countries have far more serious things to worry about than watery stools or gut ache. Perhaps the vast amount of processed and refined foods we consume in the West might give a clue as to why our bowels aren't happy.

The Asian countries, for example, have a much healthier diet, typically featuring lots of raw fish, vegetables, rice, noodles and bean curd – all freshly prepared rather than heated up in a microwave or from a packet.

Could the over-consumption of sugar, too many wheat-based products, takeaways and pre-packed foods be contributing to bowel problems like IBS in the West? It's important to consider the many different factors – the role of food is considered in chapter 9.

Could IBS be a hereditary disease?

This is a really good question – and one to which there is no simple answer. It's not possible to genetically inherit IBS but the condition can indeed run in families. Why? Stress can manifest in different ways for different people – some people might get headaches, backache, rashes or problem skin – for IBS sufferers, stress manifests in their bowels.

If one of your parents is prone to worrying or has a sensitive stomach which reacts to stress, the chances are that you will too. This doesn't suggest that IBS can be passed on through genes but rather through learned behaviour, as children may unconsciously copy their parents, relatives or friends.

Equally, if there is a family history of stress or not coping very well under pressure, this may mean that several members of the family are susceptible to stress-related IBS symptoms. Research from the Gut Trust states that parents of children with chronic, unexplained abdominal symptoms frequently have IBS themselves.

If a family eats lots of fatty, low-fibre foods, the chances are that their bowel movements are not very regular. The children in the family will probably follow the same bowel patterns if they eat the same unhealthy food. It's also possible that families could share a genetic predisposition towards certain food intolerances, but that's a different matter. There'll be more about diet and intolerances in the later chapters.

'My mum used to complain of a knotted stomach when she felt stressed. Now I'm a mother I get knotted stomachs when I worry about the kids but a hot water bottle on my belly makes it disappear!'

Jackie, Liverpool.

Action points

- Look at the food that you and your family eat. Does it include lots of fibre, fresh fruit and vegetables or is it mostly ready meals or takeaways?

- What's the typical dining pattern for you (and your family)? Do you sit down together for breakfast and dinner or do you eat separately, on the run or in front of the television? Who's the last one to finish their meal? Do you feel pressure to eat quickly so that the table can be cleared and people can get on with other things?

- Does anyone else in your immediate family suffer with IBS? Chapters 10 and 12 are packed with tips and ideas such as easily learned relaxation methods to reduce stress and adopt a more balanced attitude to life.

Summing Up

Now you know that IBS is not age discriminative – bowel problems can arise in infants, teenagers, adults and the elderly. You may be experiencing IBS due to eating an unhealthy diet or leading a stressful lifestyle, or it could even be caused from picking up habits from people around you. There are many different factors to be taken into account when determining the cause of your IBS and it's important not to blame yourself – or anyone else for that matter! The way forward is to be kind to yourself and take responsibility for what you can begin to change today for the sake of your future digestive health.

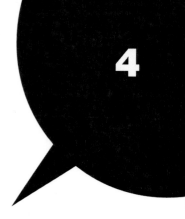

4

What Causes IBS?

The burning question is: where exactly did IBS come from and why does it affect us today when our lives are supposed to be more advanced and improved? Research has provided many explanations aiming to answer this question.

Fast-paced lives

In previous decades when men were traditionally the breadwinners and women stayed at home as full-time housewives and mothers, fresh, home-baked, seasonal cooking was all the rage. But who has the time or inclination these days for baking bread and preparing fresh sauces when you can buy it all in supermarkets or local stores, and often two for the price of one? Who would also argue that fast and convenient food makes more sense when you're juggling family life with a full-time job, dashing from daycare to meetings followed by evening deadlines – especially if you're doing it all as a single parent?

Most of us wish we could buy more time and feel that there are never enough hours in the day to get everything done, least of all the things that are fun or that we'd really love to be doing. But this pressure could be contributing to problems with our bowels.

Dietary factors

Diet is considered to be a major contributor to IBS as symptoms are often worse after eating a meal.

'Stress makes the gut sensitive, producing reactions to certain foods, and some experts believe food types like fat, alcohol, coffee and spices can make symptoms worse.'

Stress makes the gut sensitive, producing reactions to certain foods, and some experts believe food types like fat, alcohol, coffee and spices can make symptoms worse, while others believe that any food is a trigger regardless of what it is.

A high-fibre diet is considered to be the best way forward for regular and healthy bowel movements, but some forms of fibre can aggravate IBS symptoms. (See chapter 8 for more about this.)

Are you caught up in a bad cycle of eating on the go, rushing around and following a busy, hectic lifestyle? If you choose to eat food that is high on convenience but not on nutritional value, this isn't going to create a healthy digestive system.

Crisps and chocolate may be economical to buy and easy to obtain when you're in a hurry, but they're full of fat and sugar. Too much sugar can upset the gut by causing fermentation in the colon, preventing other 'feel-good' foods that you may otherwise be eating from being absorbed.

You might also be reaching for sugar-loaded cakes, biscuits or snacks to keep you going during the day, drinking too many cups of coffee or tea each day and consuming more than your fair share of alcohol each week. These are all triggers for IBS symptoms and your body can only take this overload of unhealthy foods for so long.

Common food annoyances

Food intolerances are very common today and your IBS symptoms could actually be a result of a sensitivity your body has developed towards something in your diet. It can be the other way around too – IBS and the functional problems of your digestive system are causing sensitivities to certain foods.

Food intolerances can cause bloating, diarrhoea, pain and constipation. They can occur when the body is unable to deal with certain types of food because it isn't producing enough of a particular type of enzyme or chemical to digest it. (Note that this is different to an allergy, which is when the immune system is activated.)

Intolerances can also occur if you have an inflamed gut and there are tiny lesions in the intestines, allowing food to leak into the blood and trigger a reaction. This is known as leaky gut syndrome.

Common triggers are wheat, dairy and sugars like fructose, lactose and the sweetener sorbitol. Sensitivity to lactose, fructose and sorbitol go largely undiagnosed yet they can be responsible for stomach bloating and intestinal distress in millions of people.

Your system may also be sensitive to caffeine and the array of additives used today in various products to preserve them or add colours and flavours. These include sulphites (chemicals known as E numbers E220-E228), benzoates (known as E210-E219, often found in soft drinks), monosodium glutamate, or msg (known as E621, a food additive used in Chinese cooking but also added to soups and sauces to enhance flavour), aspartame (an intense sweetener used in soft drinks and low calorie foods, known as E951) and tartrazine (known as E102, used in soft drinks, sweets and sauces).

Use the trigger diary as a tool to investigate this and consider seeing a nutritionist for some intolerance tests and dietary advice. Chapter 9 has more information on food and nutrition.

Fructose intolerance

Fructose is the sugar found in fruit and honey. Fructose-rich fruits include apples, bananas, apricots, pears, cherries, plums, prunes and peaches – plus their juices as drinks.

Some people can easily digest fructose but if you have a sensitivity to it, it can remain in the large intestine where it ferments and produces gas and bloating.

Fructose intolerance can sometimes be overlooked because wheat or dairy tend to be the most common triggers for digestive disturbance. However, researchers in the US found that 10% of people with IBS had fructose intolerance, so it's worth getting this checked out if you experience gas and bloating after eating fruit.

You can diagnose fructose intolerance via a breath test which establishes whether the breath contains hydrogen and methane. These abnormal by-products indicate that the body is not metabolising fructose normally. Talk to a nutritionist about this – see chapter 9.

'Some people can easily digest fructose but if you have a sensitivity to it, it can remain in the large intestine where it ferments and produces gas and bloating.'

When intolerance means something else

Around one in 100 people are estimated to have coeliac disease in the UK. This is a permanent intolerance to gluten, a protein found in wheat, barley and rye. If you suspect you have wheat or gluten intolerances, go to see your GP.

Lactose (the sugars found in milk/dairy) intolerance can cause symptoms that are very similar to IBS. If you suspect that milk or dairy products are triggering your symptoms, again, go and visit your GP who can establish whether you're lactose intolerant.

'My IBS was triggered when I caught a viral infection abroad. I sought advice from a nutritional therapist who prescribed anti-parasite treatment and a long dose of probiotics.'

Michelle, 38, London.

Flora imbalances/bacterial and parasitic infections

Travelling to exotic foreign climes is an extremely adventurous and enjoyable experience, but catching a nasty stomach bug is not, especially if it triggers ongoing IBS symptoms. Many people with IBS report that their symptoms started after a viral or bacterial gastroenteritis and, unfortunately, problems can persist for months or years after the infection has cleared up.

IBS could also develop after an inflammation of the stomach and bowel lining which causes sickness and diarrhoea, or after taking a continued course of antibiotics because they weaken (and destroy) much of the gut's 'good' bacteria.

Stress and emotions

The word of the times – stress – is blamed for so many illnesses, ailments and problems and is often cited to be one of the key causes of IBS – but is it really?

We all experience stress in different ways: tension headaches, sleepless nights, pimples, rashes or aches and pains. IBS symptoms are another way in which stress can manifest in us physically. Medical experts believe that stress can affect the immune system which can then trigger the onset of IBS. Stress can also make symptoms worse and increase future bouts.

Trauma

Many people report that their IBS symptoms started after a particularly stressful event or period in their life. External factors which can cause immense stress such as the death of a loved one, marital difficulties, problems with children/parents and worries related to business or education cannot be underestimated for their effect on our health.

Doctors and health experts are really coming round to the idea that IBS is caused by a malfunction of the brain-to-gut connection – if you've been through a particularly challenging time, had a shock, trauma or upset, this could be the reason why you've got IBS.

This is also the case for children. The stress of losing a parent (or both parents) or dealing with their divorce, alcoholism or drug addiction, moving to a new school or being bullied are obvious psychological factors which can trigger IBS in children and teenagers.

Can you prevent it?

This is a tough one. Because the exact cause of IBS is unknown, it's difficult to prevent IBS from developing, especially as some people are unlucky enough to develop IBS following a gut infection or food poisoning which can be near impossible to predict. However, the NHS believes symptoms can be controlled if positive lifestyle changes and treatment therapies are followed.

Since it's been proved that stress, certain foods and eating irregular meals can trigger IBS, these should be avoided if you want to prevent IBS attacks. Aiming to have a positive outlook on life, making the changes you can in order to feel happier and more relaxed are all good ways to help your bowels function less irritably and more healthily.

Generally, patients with IBS have higher levels of stress than people with other gastric disorders. However, it's a vicious circle because stress can cause IBS and IBS can cause you to feel more stressed. The trick is finding ways of breaking the cycle.

'Many people report that their IBS symptoms started after a particularly stressful event or period in their life.'

Action plan

- See if you can pinpoint when your IBS symptoms started. The point of this exercise is to see if there is any link to a long course of antibiotics, a stomach upset, food poisoning or to a particularly stressful period in your life, for example, taking GCSEs or A-levels, leaving home for the first time and going to university, starting a new job, the death of a loved one or a relationship breakdown. Identifying whether the initial trigger of the IBS was physical or psychological could help identify the best course of treatment for you.

- Refer to your IBS trigger diary and check to see if your symptoms are particularly bad on days when you've consumed particular food types, for example, lots of wheat – eating toast for breakfast, sandwiches for lunch and pasta for dinner.

- Again referring back to the IBS trigger diary, look at the days when you experienced more headaches, low moods, depression, anxiety and psychological symptoms. What happened on those days? Did you have a stressful day? What caused the stress? Did you miss your bus to school/work, have an argument or an emotional upset of some sort?

- Look for patterns. A bit of detective work needs to take place here but pattern-forming is one of the most effective ways of understanding your IBS so you can figure out how best to treat it.

Summing Up

As already highlighted in chapter 3, the exact cause of IBS is unclear and it's different for everyone. The action plan in this chapter is a great place to start answering the why, how and when questions before deciding how best to treat it. Could there be any food items that you may have overlooked, like the additives which are put into sauces, soup, wine or beer? Or are you beginning to realise that it could be less about what you eat and more about how you feel? If so, there's plenty of advice about what help is available to cope with stress and the emotional triggers in chapters 10, 11 and 12.

In the meantime, stay positive! You're on the way to avoiding, reducing and managing your IBS symptoms.

For more information on stress, see *Stress – The Essential Guide* (Need2Know).

5

IBS Symptoms

I t's now been established that IBS is a collection of symptoms rather than a single disease, and that it's the most common condition seen by gastroenterologists today.

IBS can be a painful, frustrating and embarrassing condition and it affects everyone differently. Some people can have the full house of symptoms, while others have just one or two. Some will have all of them at different times in their life. This chapter looks in detail at the many different symptoms underneath the umbrella term 'IBS'.

Typical physical IBS symptoms

- Excessive wind and burping.
- Diarrhoea.
- Constipation.
- Bad breath.

- Nausea and vomiting.

- Indigestion.

- Feeling bloated and full in the abdominal area.

- Spasms.

- Back and groin pain.

- Feeling lethargic and tired.

- Not sleeping properly and experiencing disturbed sleep patterns.

- Feeling the need to urinate more often/urgently.

This list is not exhaustive. You may also experience other problems along the gastro-intestinal (GI) tract such as heartburn, feeling as though there's something 'stuck' at the back of the throat or short, sharp stabbing pains from the rectum. This is why it's vital that you don't self-diagnose and that you visit your GP for a medical diagnosis.

Constipation

If constipation and a bloated stomach are your main symptoms, you'll have a feeling that the bowels aren't fully empty even if you have a bowel movement every day. You may also feel that your breath smells. If you can't go to the toilet for days at a time, you'll have to strain more than is good for you and your stools will be hard and lumpy.

Diarrhoea

If diarrhoea is the predominant symptom, food will pass through your digestive system faster than normal. Diarrhoea is often usually associated with being on the continent or eating some dodgy prawns, but if the diarrhoea continues for some time then it's chronic and could be a symptom of IBS.

Abdominal pain

Some people experience sharp, gripping central abdominal cramps and/or pain on either the right or the lower left of the abdomen, sometimes so bad that their professional and social appointments need to be cancelled. The pain might improve or worsen by going to the toilet, passing wind or eating.

Bloating, swelling and squeaking noises

Bowel contents are moved along by a series of rhythms which tighten and relax segments of the intestine, a process called peristalsis. The peristalsis motions are stronger and noisier in IBS sufferers and cause abdominal rumblings as gases are moved though the intestines. Sufferers also feel bloated, windy and uncomfortable.

The psychological symptoms

Do you often feel nervous, sometimes for no rational or apparent reason? Do you have trouble sleeping, often waking up and worrying about things like exams, work meetings or arguments with members of the family, friends or your partner? Or do you suffer with tension headaches, low moods or depression? These are all noted IBS symptoms.

According to the NHS, up to 60% of people with IBS experience psychological symptoms such as anxiety and depression and studies suggest that IBS is caused by a disorder in the brain-to-gut connection. Studies have also shown that IBS sufferers tend to have a lower threshold for coping with stressful situations in life which can negatively impact their digestive system. So, as you can see, it's a bit of a vicious circle but it can be broken. There's more about this in the following chapters.

Typical psychological IBS symptoms

- Headaches.
- Nervousness.
- Heightened stress levels.
- Depression.
- Anxiety.
- Panicky feelings.

However, because some of the IBS symptoms can mimic other digestive disorders, it's not always clear if someone has IBS. If you recognise any of the following 'red flag' symptoms in addition to the typical IBS symptoms, it's recommended that you make an appointment to see your GP to discuss them.

'Patients prone to anxiety or depression are more susceptible to IBS than those who are not.'

Dr Suneil Kapadia, consultant gastroenterologist at New Cross Hospital, Royal Wolverhampton NHS Trust.

Red flag symptoms

- Bleeding from the rectum.

- Blood with the stools.

- Indigestion-type pain that keeps you awake at night.

- Weight loss.

- Anaemia.

- Being over 45 and having a family history of cancer or inflammatory bowel disease (IBD).

Action points

Use the table opposite to tick the symptoms you've suffered with persistently in the past three months. This is not meant to be a diagnostic test but it will help you to notice which symptoms you've got and the frequency in which they occur.

If you tick two or more symptoms, you may have IBS, but if you also have symptoms that appear on the red flag list then make an appointment to see your GP today to rule out any other serious illnesses.

Symptoms	Often	Sometimes	Never
Constipation			
Diarrhoea			
Abdominal pain			
Urgent need to 'go'			
Excessive wind			
Bloated stomach			
Headaches			
Irritability			
Depression			
Anxiety			
Dizziness			
Mood swings			
Insomnia			

Summing Up

From this chapter it's easy to see why IBS is called a mysterious disease! The condition comes in many different disguises and no two people experience IBS in the same way. The symptom checklist will certainly help you establish which symptoms are most common for you, but remember these can change at any time, new ones can appear and others may disappear then re-emerge at another time. As already stated in the previous chapters, you'll need to establish what triggers your symptoms, however it is vitally important that you get properly diagnosed. Turn to chapter 6 for more information about the IBS diagnosis process.

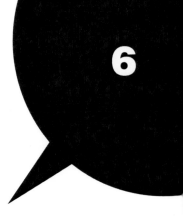

6

Being Diagnosed

I f you suspect that you (or someone close to you) have IBS, it's vital that you go and see your GP for a medical diagnosis. Making an appointment to visit your GP to talk about your bowel movements may feel daunting – you might feel anxious about what will happen and how they will establish your condition, or have deeper concerns that something more serious will be discovered.

Whatever you feel, it's really important to go and talk to a health professional rather than leaving things in the vain hope that they will go away.

When should you go and see your GP?

There isn't a standard answer to this question. Some health professionals say that if you have recurring symptoms for three months you should seek medical guidance. Others recommend seeking medical advice as soon as you notice a change in your bowel patterns.

However, our bowel habits often change while we're away on holiday due to a different diet/environment or before/during/after a big event – we're creatures of habit and the slightest thing can disrupt our rhythms.

Usually things settle down quickly once back in a routine. But if you're worried, go and see you GP – don't feel you need to wait a set amount of time.

Getting tested

Unfortunately there isn't one single method to diagnose IBS, but the good news is that it takes much less time than it used to.

Previously, doctors would perform various tests to rule out more serious conditions and check there was nothing more sinister than IBS. This was hard for the patient, first having to go through the discomfort of the tests then playing the waiting game, which would invariably add to any stress-related symptoms until the results arrived.

This is no longer the case, so if you've been suffering with IBS symptoms for some time and have been hoping the symptoms will clear up or disappear, it's time to go and get things checked out. The sooner you do so, the sooner your condition can be confirmed and you can move on and find an appropriate treatment.

'You may feel uncomfortable and embarrassed talking about your bowel movements, but this is necessary for the doctor to make a proper diagnosis.'

Seeing your GP about IBS

GPs generally diagnose IBS by a process of elimination. It's a case of looking at what symptoms a person has and what they don't have. When you go to see your doctor, tell him/her all about your symptoms and how long you've had them for. If it helps, make a list before you go and take your trigger diary or any questions or notes you've made. Your GP will look at your medical history and lifestyle to rule out any other possibly important causes of the symptoms. He/she will also ask about your diet and have a feel of your abdomen, especially if one of your symptoms is abdominal pain. They will ask you about the type of pain you experience, when it comes on and if anything makes it worse (triggers it) or if anything helps to ease it.

You may feel uncomfortable and embarrassed talking about your bowel movements and the colour, shape and size of your stools, but this is necessary for the doctor to make a proper diagnosis.

If you're under the age of 40, doctors are more likely to diagnose IBS if you have some of the typical symptoms. He/she will suggest ways of treating the symptoms, for example with a fibre supplement for constipation or peppermint oil tablets to help relax the bowels and reduce abdominal pain. (Chapter 8 covers treatments in detail.)

Seeing a gastroenterologist about IBS

After discussing your symptoms with your GP, he/she may decide that more clarification is needed or you may feel you need more reassurance that there isn't anything serious happening. In this case they may refer you to a gastroenterologist (or a gynaecologist if you're a woman experiencing IBS symptoms like abdominal pain during your period – see chapter 7).

When you see a gastroenterologist, your appointment time will be longer and more specialised than with your GP. You may want to ask a supportive friend or family member to accompany you.

Ruling out other illnesses

Sometimes IBS symptoms can mimic other serious disorders, such as:

- Bowel cancer. This is considered to be uncommon under the age of 40, but its incidence increases as we become older. As with all cancers, early diagnosis is vital.

- Inflammatory bowel disease (IBD) and Crohn's disease. These conditions can cause inflammation of any part of the gastro-intestinal tract. Ulcerative colitis involves inflammation and ulceration of the rectum and colon.

- Coeliac disease. This is caused by intolerance to gluten (a protein found in grains like wheat, rye, oats and barley) which destroys the lining of the bowel. Symptoms can appear very similar to IBS because fats and other nutrients aren't being absorbed properly. Your GP can do a blood test or a small bowel biopsy. Treatment is a strict gluten-free diet.

'A detailed assessment leading to a diagnosis of IBS will often allow you to move forwards with a treatment plan.'

Dr Suneil Kapadia, consultant gastroenterologist at New Cross Hospital, Royal Wolverhampton NHS Trust.

Interview with Dr Suneil Kapadia, consultant gastroenterologist at New Cross Hospital, Royal Wolverhampton NHS Trust.

'In the consultation I ask a whole range of questions, including about what's happening in a patient's life. It's very much a case of assessing the patient as a whole and not their symptoms in isolation. Major events such as having a baby, losing someone close, getting married or being made redundant can have a major impact on the functioning of the bowel. Patients often think it's all about what's happening in their tummies, and it doesn't occur to them that the way they're feeling and their stress levels could actually be causing digestive problems.

There is no single investigation to diagnose IBS but nevertheless there are important tests (usually blood tests) that need to be done. The condition varies from person to person but IBS does seem to affect women more, and is found in many countries.

I find that a significant part of treating IBS is spending time with the patient to enable them to understand what's actually going on in their digestive system. One of the most important things is to reassure patients that their symptoms are consistent with IBS and, although very troublesome, are not due to something more serious such as cancer.

In my experience, a thorough explanation goes a long way to treating someone with IBS. Some patients will not require any specific therapy, whereas others will need to start some form of medication depending on their predominant symptom.'

Diagnostic tests

If your GP thinks that your IBS is caused by an infection, you will be asked to give a sample of your faeces which will be sent to a laboratory for testing.

If you have unusual symptoms such as losing weight or passing blood in your faeces, your GP may want to do extra tests. He/she may want to refer you to the hospital for further tests if you have a family history of bowel problems, are over 45 and have recently developed IBS for the first time or if you have diarrhoea-only IBS. This is because these symptoms can be linked to other bowel conditions.

Any of the following investigations may be carried out and if no obvious abnormality is found, IBS is usually diagnosed.

- A stool test.

- An X-ray of your abdomen such as a barium enema. Liquid containing a small amount of barium is passed through a tube into your back passage where it enters the large intestine. The barium allows inflamed or ulcerated areas of the colon to show up clearly in X-ray images.

- An ultrasound – a procedure which uses high-frequency sound waves to view internal organs and produce images of the human body.

- A gastroscopy – a small camera attached to a thin tube (endoscope) examines the oesophagus, stomach and small intestine to see if there is any damage.

- A colonoscopy – an endoscope may be used to look inside your bowel. This is called a sigmoidoscopy or colonoscopy, depending on the part of your bowel that your doctor needs to look at.

- A biopsy may need to be taken. This involves removing a small piece of tissue from the bowel lining for examination in a laboratory. This test helps to rule out conditions such as ulcerative colitis.

Summing Up

Going to see your GP and gaining an understanding of the condition goes a long way to treating your IBS and, as Dr Suneil Kapadia confirms, there's no right or wrong time to go and see your GP. Put simply, if you're worried, pick up the phone and make an appointment. Once you do you'll probably wonder why you didn't do it sooner. However, if after your appointment you don't feel reassured, or feel that your GP didn't explain things very well or answer all of your questions, ask to be referred to a gastroenterologist where there will be more time to voice your concerns with someone who is a specialist in this part of the body. Once IBS is diagnosed there are many different treatment options to consider. You'll learn all about these in the following chapters.

7

Women and IBS

This chapter is dedicated to women due to the collective belief that the female population tends to experience IBS more than men and that it often affects them differently.

This chapter explores ways for women to improve and reduce symptoms, highlighting the importance of relaxation and diet modification to reduce bloating, along with other psychological measures to feel more positive and in control of their IBS.

Is it really true?

Chapter 3 looked at the figures and research which suggest that IBS affects women more than men. The NHS cites IBS as being twice as common in women than men and the UK Charity, IBS Research Appeal, reports that a staggering three times more women are likely to be seen in their clinics than men. (In one of their Bristol clinics 75–80% of consulters were also female.)

It's been suggested that IBS could be more prevalent in women because they have more sensitive guts and because food has a psychological significance for them. Traditionally, men regard food as fuel to provide energy but, then again, many men are foodies and passionately into gastronomy!

Menstruation and IBS

'Abdominal pains and/or pain during sex can occur in patients with IBS symptoms but they could also point to a gynaecological problem which may also need to be explored.'

Dr Suneil Kapadia, consultant gastroenterologist at New Cross Hospital, Royal Wolverhampton NHS Trust.

Women often experience changes in their bowel habits during their menstrual cycle. For many women, IBS symptoms become much worse. They may need to go to the toilet more frequently (even if normally constipated) or experience an increase in gas, abdominal pain and maybe even diarrhoea. This is usually attributed to hormonal fluctuations, i.e. the changing levels of oestrogen and progesterone.

However, studies show that the approximate amount of time for contents to move from the mouth to the rectum is the same regardless of the time in the month. This suggests that the physical symptoms of IBS are more likely exacerbated around the time of a woman's period because of things like a change in diet (for example, craving more chocolate, sugar or alcohol before a period) or increased stress, tension and anxiety (otherwise known as PMS).

Gynaecological check-ups

According to Dr Suneil Kapadia, consultant gastroenterologist at New Cross Hospital, Royal Wolverhampton NHS Trust, a range of possibilities needs to be taken into account when diagnosing IBS in women. Your GP may want to refer you to a gynaecologist if you experience painful sex or abdominal pains. Although these can be typical IBS symptoms, they could indicate a gynaecological problem which should be explored in greater detail. So, if you experience regular abdominal pain or pain during sex, it's advisable that you discuss them with your GP so that they can be fully investigated.

Positive ways to avoid stress-induced IBS symptoms

Diaries and (a little bit of) chocolate

Keeping a diary is a great way of keeping track of when you can expect your period and to adjust your diet and social life accordingly. The National Association for Premenstrual Syndrome is a helpful resource with an online diary tool to help you keep track of when your period is due and note symptoms as they occur. The website to visit is www.pms.org.uk.

It goes without saying that eating a balanced diet and avoiding foods which can make PMS or IBS symptoms worse is preferable, and the need for relaxation at this time is all the more important. If you feel more wind and gas symptoms, modify your diet, for example by reducing gas-producing foods such as cauliflower, broccoli and onions. Another useful resource for IBS and PMS is the Natural Health Advisory Service (formerly called the Women's Nutritional Advisory Service). Their website is packed with information about conquering IBS and PMS through a healthy diet and complementary therapies. You can visit the Natural Health Advisory Service at www.naturalhealthas.com.

If you crave chocolate and sugary snacks like cakes and biscuits before your period, try to swap them for healthier alternatives. Agave syrup is a good sugar substitute which is preferable to sugar or artificial sweeteners – it's a plant-derived syrup without any calories which is good for keeping blood sugar levels on an even keel. Check your supermarket or health food shop.

Anyone experiencing sugar cravings will know how hard it is to quit (myself included), but at the end of the day you have to weigh up the pros and cons. Do you want that short term sugar or chocolate hit or do you want to feel better and avoid that bloated and miserable feeling during your period?

However, certain schools of thought say that chocolate (particularly dark chocolate) is good for you – if a few squares of dark chocolate help you sail through the day then go for it!

'If you crave chocolate and sugary snacks like cakes and biscuits before your period, try to swap them for healthier alternatives. Agave syrup is a good sugar substitute.'

Saying 'no'

Sometimes we put up with things rather than rock the boat because it feels safer and less stressful at the time. But if you find yourself always saying 'yes' to people's demands such as your boss asking you to stay late, and not being able to say 'no' to a neighbour's request for favours like collecting their children from school, you will begin to feel worn down.

Practise saying 'no'. This doesn't have to be aggressive – you can be perfectly pleasant and nice about it. Try: 'No, I'm sorry but I won't be able to collect your children from school,' or 'We'd love to join you on the sailing trip on Saturday but we've got other plans – I do hope you ask me again in the future.' Buy a book about assertive communication or look for a course or workshop near you.

Wonder woman

There is tremendous pressure on women today to be a super mum or wonder woman, both totally unrealistic goals. If you've got a high-powered and stressful job, you might feel guilty about neglecting your family by working long hours. You may also feel overwhelmed by all the household chores and things that need to be done for a smooth-running family life.

Again, if you're working in a job which is unsatisfying or boring but necessary for financial reasons, it could also be having a negative impact on your life. Boring jobs where we don't feel stretched, utilised or fully appreciated can be as bad for our mental health as those which are highly demanding.

Single mums have a tremendous amount to deal with and have little (or no) time for themselves as they put their children's needs before their own, often neglecting their own diet, feeling too exhausted at the end of the day to eat. Over time, going without proper, healthy meals or eating badly due to lack of time or preparation will have a negative impact on the digestive system and your health.

Overwhelm

Many women feel they have a whole list of things to do once the working day is finished, for example planning and preparing meals, shopping and organising household things, helping with fancy dress costumes or the children's extra-curricular activities.

Guilt overwhelm may be a regular feeling when there doesn't ever seem to be enough time in the day, but high stress levels won't help the digestive system. There's more about managing stress and delegating tasks in chapters 10 and 12. Meanwhile, below are some suggestions to try.

Action points

- Write down what causes you to feel stressed, whether it's due to a relationship with your partner, parents or boss, or if it's feeling bored or over-pressurised in your current job, at college or school.

- Consider what (if anything) can be changed by some action on your part.

- Get hold of a book about assertion, such as Gael Lindenfield's *Assert Yourself* (Thorsons), which lists our basic human rights and is packed with tips on how to be assertive. This could result in motivating you to delegate household chores if you feel like no one is helping you!

- Consider how your thoughts or attitudes could be affecting how you feel and behave, thereby altering your digestive system. Cognitive behaviour therapy (CBT) is a very effective talking therapy with a great success rate – there's more about this in chapter 8.

- Give yourself permission to enjoy some time for yourself each day to kick back and listen to some music, read a book or magazine, see friends for a gossip or to indulge in a candlelit bath with a few drops of relaxing aromatherapy oils.

- Block out some time for relaxation during your period when your IBS symptoms could be heightened due to PMS/hormonal changes or sugar cravings. Consider taking up a yoga class or an interest which you would find relaxing.

'Guilt overwhelm may be a regular feeling when there doesn't ever seem to be enough time in the day, but high stress levels won't help the digestive system.'

Summing Up

Stay positive and motivated by reminding yourself on a daily basis of all the things you achieve throughout the day – at work, in your family/home or in your personal life – but let yourself off the hook if you succumb to scoffing a whole pack of biscuits or snap at your partner/colleague/kids! Although it can feel uncomfortable, especially if things feel deep-rooted and your routine is set in stone, be brave! It takes time, determination and perseverance to make changes in your life, but it's worth trying something new to see if it makes a positive impact on your IBS and stress levels. Good luck!

8

Treating Your IBS

There are many different IBS treatment options – from dietary and nutritional advice, prescriptive or over-the-counter medicines to talking therapies like counselling and psychotherapy.

Below are some of the conventional medicines available for some of the key symptoms. Note that these are for information only and should not be taken without the advice of your GP.

Mostly constipation, wind and bloating

Constipation can make you feel utterly miserable and it can take a few months of treatment before a regular bowel pattern can be re-established. GPs often recommend fibre supplements which can be bought over the counter.

Fybogel, Isogel, Celevac and Normacol are bulk-forming laxatives containing Ispaghula husk, a form of soluble fibre that increases the volume of the gut contents, helping the muscle in the gut to push the contents along more quickly.

Some people have alternating diarrhoea and constipation and Celevac (Methylcellulose) is recommended for both because it's a bulking agent and can add bulk to the stool for diarrhoea sufferers or make stools softer and easier to pass if constipated.

The right kind of fibre

Your GP may tell you to eat more fibre to relieve constipation symptoms, but you need to make sure it's the 'right' kind of fibre! There are two types: 'insoluble' and 'soluble'.

Ironically, insoluble fibre can (and rather confusingly!) often make symptoms of flatulence and wind worse as they are less digestible than soluble fibres. You may have noticed in your IBS trigger diary that certain fibre-rich foods worsen or improve your IBS. Insoluble fibres include wheat bran, wholegrain breads and cereals, wholemeal bread/cereals/pasta, lentils, fibrous vegetables (including starchy carbohydrates like potatoes), oats, barley and fruit. Insoluble fibre is often referred to as 'roughage', meaning fruit and vegetables with their skins on.

The friendlier fibre, if you like, is the soluble type which includes soft vegetables like carrots, peas, parsnips, spinach, chickpeas, butter beans and grains like quinoa or buckwheat. These can help the bowel regain health, minus any embarrassing wind or gas!

Mostly diarrhoea symptoms

If your trigger diary highlights certain foods or drinks that cause or worsen your symptoms, then reducing these is a preferred method of treating diarrhoea. Stimulants like tea, coffee and alcohol are guaranteed to worsen your symptoms. It's really important to drink lots of fresh water each day (at least two litres per day) to help replace bodily fluids and prevent dehydration.

You can buy anti-diarrhoeal tablets like Imodium over the counter which help to reduce the frequency of bowel movements by slowing down intestinal muscular contractions. However, if your symptoms are so bad that you can't leave the house for fear of an accident, this will undoubtedly be making you feel very isolated, not to mention depressed. As a result, antidepressants are often prescribed by GPs to treat some of the IBS symptoms like diarrhoea, pain and depression because they increase feel-good chemicals to the brain and help to reduce pain. The most commonly prescribed tablets are called 'tricyclics', or TCAs. Some names include amitriptyline, clomipramine, doxepin and trimipramine.

However, there are plenty of alternatives to antidepressants that can help with the psychological or emotional aspects of IBS (see the following chapters) and are more empowering and preferable to those who want to avoid taking pills.

Mostly abdominal pains

For many IBS sufferers, abdominal pains can be so excruciating that all social or professional appointments have to be cancelled. The pain can come on quite suddenly, so if you're at home it's much easier to lay down with a hot water bottle on your belly until the pain subsides!

You GP may recommend some anti-spasmodic tablets which can help relax the muscles in your bowels. Some names include Mebeverine (Colofac IBS), Alverine (Spasmonal), Hyoscine (Buscopan) and Dicycloverine (Merbentyl).

Peppermint oil tablets are another time-proven formula which can help relax the muscles in the bowels and reduce colonic contractility and pain. They are quite reasonable in price and available over the counter. Peppermint tea can also be good but the tablets are deemed more effective.

Recent studies led by gastroenterologist Dr Alex Ford (from the gastroenterology division at McMaster University in Ontario) concluded that peppermint oil is the top IBS treatment, along with the anti-spasmodic Hyoscine and soluble fibre.

If abdominal pain is a regular occurrence and you are female, your GP may want to do some further investigations to rule out other gynaecological conditions (see chapters 6 and 7).

'My GP prescribed peppermint oil tablets for my abdominal pain and constipation, but the strong flavour kept repeating on me. I tried reflexology, and after six sessions my symptoms have disappeared!'

Lisa, former IBS sufferer.

Complementary therapies

Complementary therapies have been found to be highly effective in treating IBS as they're particularly good at helping a person deal with stress and anxiety, as well as encouraging the body to heal itself.

Some of the most popular are acupuncture, aromatherapy massage, reflexology and hypnotherapy, but there are plenty more and the following list is not exhaustive.

Acupuncture

A practitioner inserts very fine needles into your skin at specific points to reduce pain and other symptoms. Acupuncture works on the premise that disease or disharmony occurs in the body when energy or 'Qi' is blocked. The needles are positioned in strategic places on the body to stimulate the body's own healing response, remove blockages and restore, promote and maintain good health. There are almost 3,000 qualified acupuncturists registered with the British Acupuncture Council today – visit www.acupuncture.org.uk for more information.

Aromatherapy

Aromatherapy essential oils have many psychological and physiological benefits: reducing illness, relieving anxiety, exhaustion, depression and stress and promoting relaxation – all good things for IBS sufferers. Aromatherapy is a holistic treatment combining the healing touch of massage with therapeutic scents which impact the central nervous system. Essential oils are extracted from plants, flowers, trees, fruits, bark, grasses and seeds. You can enjoy a professional aromatherapy massage or buy oils for DIY treatment. You could add two drops of lavender (or geranium, bergamot and sandalwood) oil to a teaspoon of sweet almond oil and place it in a burner for an uplifting aroma in your home or add it to your bath.

Herbalism

For centuries, herbs and plants have been used for their therapeutic value. They produce and contain a variety of chemical compounds which can be used on the body to prevent/treat disease or promote health and wellbeing. There are three main branches of herbalism: Indian Ayurveda, Chinese herbal medicine and Greek/Roman/Medieval sources. Ayurveda originated in India some 5,000 years ago and can teach you to eat correctly for your 'dosha' (personality/constitution). For example, fiery, energetic people who fall under the 'Pitta' dosha should avoid hot, spicy foods and caffeine as their system is more sensitive to these stimulants. A useful resource is the College of Ayurveda website (www.ayurvedacollege.org.uk). Ethnobotanist James Wong recently presented a programme on BBC2 called *Grow Your Own Drugs* to show us how to heal our ailments through herbs and plants. See www.bbc.co.uk/programmes/b00j3ktd for more information on the programme.

Homeopathy

This is a gentle and holistic healing system, treating like for like in a similar way to a vaccination, except that homeopathy is completely natural. Pills are made from plants and minerals to boost the body's defence mechanisms which work on the individual as a whole, taking into account not just physical symptoms but emotional ones as well. There are several antidepressant formulas like Ignatia Amara, or Pulsatilla, which offer a more natural alternative to prescriptive TCAs. Contact the Society of Homeopaths at www.homeopathy-soh.org for more information.

Naturopathy

This refers to a holistic system of medicine drawing on nature's healing powers. Naturopaths seek the cause of disease by understanding the patient as a whole, finding the underlying cause whether it is physical, mental or emotional, and using nutrition, herbal medicine, homeopathy and acupuncture.

Reflexology

Reflexologists press on different points of the feet to stimulate a beneficial effect on the various organs and systems of the body. Working on the premise that the foot is divided into a number of reflex zones corresponding to zones of energy in the body, therapists apply pressure to the various points of a person's foot to stimulate the corresponding part of the body to prompt self-healing. This is renowned for improving digestive health and IBS symptoms. Visit www.aor.org.uk for more information.

Other natural ways to treat IBS

Eating

What you eat, how you eat and when you eat plays a large part in treating your IBS, especially if you suspect food intolerances are involved. There's more about food and diet in chapter 9.

Exercise

The gut is a muscle which needs exercising. Any exercise is good for your digestion and a brisk walk before eating is a great way to maintain healthy bowel movements.

'The gut is a muscle which needs exercising. Any exercise is good for your digestion and a brisk walk before eating is a great way to maintain healthy bowel movements.'

Inner cleansing

Some people swear by colonics, yet others are horrified at the very thought of having a tube attached to their bottom! Colonic irrigation (also known as colonic hydrotherapy) removes toxins and waste from the bowels by cleansing the large intestine with warm water.

The water circulates around the colon (the large intestine) to stimulate the bowel to empty. This is considered very effective for constipation, bloating, diarrhoea and removing parasites.

Yoga

Yoga can be a tremendous therapy for IBS. The many different postures (asanas) stretch and massage the internal organs and have a very beneficial and rejuvenating effect on the body's systems. Specific postures which aid the digestive system can be learned as well as relaxation techniques which can help with stress (these can even be practised in bed to help promote quality sleep).

There are many different styles of yoga but for stress-related IBS a gentle Hatha yoga class (rather than dynamic or hot yoga) is recommended. I trained in Sivananda, a branch of Hatha, which focuses on regular and systematic practice of postures to help stimulate, improve and maintain good health (www.sivananda.org). Check your area for yoga classes or visit the British Wheel of Yoga's website for a list of accredited teachers around the country (www.bwy.org.uk).

The talking therapies

Pessimistic thoughts can cause stress and anxiety and could be causing or adding to your IBS symptoms. The talking therapies like counselling, psychotherapy and cognitive behaviour therapy (CBT) can help you understand the emotional symptoms of IBS. You will get the opportunity to learn new ways of dealing with stressful or negative thoughts and feelings by turning them into more positive ones.

Counselling and psychotherapy

Counsellors are usually qualified to diploma level and trained to help you explore your thoughts and feelings and alter negative beliefs. Psychotherapists usually have a postgraduate qualification in psychotherapy, but both can help with anxiety, depression, mood swings and low self-esteem which could be affecting your IBS.

Your GP may refer you to see a counsellor on the NHS, but if there's a really long waiting list you may decide to go privately – visit the British Association for Counselling and Psychotherapy online (www.bacp.co.uk) to find a reputable practitioner.

Admittedly, private therapy can be expensive but there are several charities – BACP can tell you about low-cost counselling schemes which are available to students, people on low incomes and the unemployed. Some companies offer their staff (and sometimes family members) an employee assistance counselling scheme – check with your employer's Human Resources department.

Cognitive behaviour therapy (CBT)

'Cognitive' means the way you think about yourself and how you perceive the world around you. This therapy allows you step back and look at how you're behaving in relation to the things that are happening in your life. It allows you to learn how to change your negative thinking. CBT is becoming much more readily available on the NHS – ask your GP about it or take a proactive approach in the *Feeling Good Handbook* (Plume) by David D. Burns, MD.

Hypnotherapy

This is an extremely popular and very effective therapy for IBS due to the link between the nervous system, the brain and the gut – see chapter 11. Hypnotherapy can help you manage symptoms like sleeping problems, panic attacks, anxiety and stress, as well as the physical symptoms, through mind-over-matter techniques. The hypnotherapist uses 'suggestion' to train the patient's subconscious mind to adopt productive ways of managing stress and anxiety. A number of studies suggest that hypnosis can successfully help patients gain control over their digestive systems. It has shown to be especially effective for women.

'Hypnotherapy is really beneficial if you find it impossible to relax. The hypnotherapist's instructions bypass the expectations of the patient's conscious mind, allowing the unconscious mind to respond in a new way.'

Cat Murphy, Hypnotherapist, Brighton.

Summing Up

You don't need to make a choice between conventional (allopathic) medicine and complementary (alternative) therapies because they work well alongside each other. However, you must always keep your therapist/GP informed about which treatment(s) you're having. If you haven't already done so, it's worth trying some of the over-the-counter medicines mentioned to treat wind, abdominal pain, constipation or diarrhoea to see if they're beneficial to you. Making a simple change to the type of fibre you eat or increasing the amount of exercise you take could equally very quickly have effective results.

Prices for complementary and talking therapies vary – expect to pay in the region of £30 for an hour's treatment (depending on your location). Some therapy centres offer promotional deals or taster sessions so you can sample them at much lower prices. If possible, get a personal recommendation and always ask about the therapist's qualifications/training. If your body is particularly responsive to the therapy you may feel the results immediately, but it generally takes some time to see the positive benefits. Many complementary therapists say that you'll often feel worse before you can feel better – so commitment and perseverance are absolutely essential!

Food and Nutrition

Which foods should I avoid?

n an ideal world there would be a compilation of foods to avoid if you had IBS, but studies suggest that one person's food can be another person's poison.

IBS Research Appeal questioned IBS sufferers about which foods were helpful and which weren't. They found that items like citrus fruits, alcohol, cereals and milk were on both lists, adding to the view that no two people experience IBS in the same way.

Fatty, spicy and sugary foods are generally thought to be unhelpful in our diets, and processed foods are more likely to cause problems than natural products.

The most common IBS triggers tend to be cow's milk and wheat. Although we can digest these without any issue from an early age, the digestive system is less able to cope as we grow older and intolerances can develop.

What the gut needs for smooth digestion

It's not just about what you eat, but how and when you eat it. If you're always on the go, eating breakfast on the way to work or school, gobbling lunch at your desk or grabbing a burger on the train home, then it's time to rethink your dining routine.

At the Viva Mayr health resort in Carinthia, Austria, a centre for digestive health, traditional and naturopathic treatments are practised based on the concepts of an Austrian physician, Dr F. X. Mayr (1875–1965).

The focus is on strict cleansing of the digestive system and the reform of eating habits; slowing down and chewing food properly to encourage proper

digestion and optimal nutrition. The resort treats a whole range of disorders including IBS, food intolerances, backache and fertility problems by cleansing and regenerating the digestive system.

According to Dr Harald Stossier, Medical Director at the Viva Mayr in Austria, the reason so many of us have digestive problems today is because we're not chewing food properly, we're eating it too fast, too late in the evening and drowning it with soft sugary drinks or wine.

Rhythms

Due to modern lifestyles most of us eat our main meal in the evening, going against the natural rhythm of our bodies. Dr Harald Stossier believes that good digestive health can be achieved by developing a rhythm in life – eating the right kind of food at the right time of day and chewing it efficiently.

Our digestive systems function better in the morning. This is also the time when our energy levels are the highest. Mayr medicine states that this is when the system can cope with digestion better and when you should eat more, taking the main meal of the day at lunchtime and a light meal (like soup and bread) in the early evening.

Because the body's metabolism slows down after 2pm, the body is less able to digest raw salads or heavily processed salty, sugary or fatty foods after this time. Eating late in the evening overloads the digestive system, preventing it from regenerating at night.

'It's essential to eat in the right way, to chew food properly (at least 50 times) and avoid drinking with your meal which prevents the digestive juices from working efficiently.'

Dr Harald Stossier, medical director, the Viva Mayr Health Resort, Austria.

Mucus

The digestive tract is normally coated with a layer of mucus which helps to keep out foreign substances. Having a strong lining of mucus is really important for healthy digestion. Leaky gut syndrome can develop if the mucus layer is weakened and bacteria from the intestines move to other parts of the body (this is known as bacterial translocation).

If you're dehydrated or stressed, this lining of mucus can become thin and cause digestive problems. However, you can help to repair the lining and maintain the mucus with various supplements.

According to Susie Perry, a nutritional therapist from East Sussex, taking concentrated Aloe Vera juice for one to three months will help restore the lining of mucus in the gut. Concentrated Aloe Vera juice is available in large chemists like Boots. If you've got a cactus plant at home, you could squeeze the leaf and take a teaspoon of the juice to drink.

Slippery Elm or Marshmallow herb capsules can soothe an acidic and inflamed gut. Turmeric is also a renowned and powerful anti-inflammatory agent that treats inflammation of the gut at the microscopic level. Try taking a 500 or 1,000 milligram capsule each day or use it in your cooking.

The Indian spice Asafoetida is considered beneficial for digestion and is a good alternative to onions or garlic which can cause flatulence for some people (it even tastes a little like garlic). Peppermint is also really good for digestion and mint can easily be incorporated to your cooking – see Susie Perry's sample menus at the end of the chapter.

Adding ginger or cinnamon to a glass of hot water can also smooth the digestive process, as can herbal teas like chamomile, ginger, fennel and peppermint.

An abundance of friendly bacteria

It's really important to have lots of good, friendly bacteria in the gut. There are many different types of probiotic and bio ('good' bacteria) yogurt-type drinks on the market which claim to keep the digestive system healthy (especially important if you've recently taken a course of antibiotics or had a gut infection as the friendly bacteria will be strongly diminished).

However, probiotic supplements are more effective because there are millions of friendly bacteria in just one tablet – you'd have to eat a lot of yogurt to get the same result (look for the tablets which have one billion cells per dose). BioCare is a trusted brand for supplements and is available online.

The right combination of foods

Nutrition isn't just about food, it's also about the digestion of food. Any food can be the 'wrong' food if eaten very late in the day, in a hurry or in the wrong combination!

According to Dr Stossier at the Viva Mayr, digestive conditions like IBS or leaky gut syndrome can be caused by eating too many acidic-type foods which imbalance the digestive system. Many nutritionists and digestive experts favour the food combining theory which involves eating chemically compatible food to allow the body to digest more efficiently.

Food combining means not eating protein such as beans, meat and fish with starches like pasta, bread or rice (proteins and starchy carbohydrates are both acidic foods and together they are not so digestible). Try combining fish, cheese or meat with salad or vegetables and potatoes (even though potatoes are a starchy carbohydrate they're very alkaline and very good for the system) for lunch, then a vegetable soup for dinner.

See the sample menu compiled by the Chef at the Viva Mayr Resort at the end of the chapter which is an example of protein food combining and involves salmon (protein) with vegetables rather than rice or pasta. Food combining may not be for everyone, but it's worth trying it to see if your IBS symptoms improve.

'Nutrition isn't just about food, it's also about the digestion of food. Any food can be the 'wrong' food if eaten very late in the day, in a hurry or in the wrong combination!'

The nutritionist's approach to IBS

Nutritionists and nutritional therapists advise clients about healthy diets, recommend supplements, perform food allergy testing and give advice about detoxing, colon health, digestion and absorption.

Nutritional therapists and nutritionists are trained to look for the underlying causes of health problems, applying their clinical skills to create a personalised programme which addresses specific issues and helps you reach your health goals.

Using various tests they can find out what nutrients and vitamins a person is low in and devise a healthy nutrition plan.

Interview with Susie Perry, a nutritional therapist.

'The first thing I do is establish whether I think a person has classic IBS or a digestive disturbance. If I suspect IBS I refer them to their GP for a medical diagnosis.

'I ask questions about their diet, health and lifestyle, and if it's obvious that the diet is out of balance, I'll go down the dietary treatment route.

'It's basically an elimination process – I'll ask my client to write down everything they've eaten in the past seven days. I'll be looking for how much wheat, gluten, citrus, yeast and dairy has been consumed. I can test for nutritional, biochemical, hormonal and toxic factors, from parasites to thyroid function with a saliva, blood, urine or stool test, and I use one of Europe's leading diagnostic laboratories.

'If a woman's IBS symptoms are worse mid-cycle, I'll do some hormonal explorations. If symptoms occur when the client goes to a meeting or before a speech at work, I'll do some stress investigations, then help them work on self-esteem and stress management.

'I've noticed after 10 years of practice that alcohol and sugar, singularly or together, can heighten intolerances and greatly impact the digestive system's functioning.

'Patients generally need a minimum of between three and four sessions, dependent on test results (if taken).'

Consultation charges vary – expect to pay in the region of £60 for the first consultation, depending on location.

The Nutritional Therapy Council is the governing body for nutritionists in the UK.

You can go to the British Association for Applied Nutrition and Nutritional Therapy (BANT) website to locate a qualified therapist near you (www.bant.org.uk).

'Nutrition is a holistic therapy – it's not just about looking at how much fibre someone has in their gut.'

Susie Perry, nutritional therapist and founder of Nurturing Spirit, her nutritional therapy company in East Sussex.

Testing for intolerances

Food intolerances can occur when the body is unable to deal with certain types of food because it isn't producing enough of a particular type of enzyme or chemical to digest it. (Note that this is different to an allergy, which is when the immune system is activated.) Common triggers are wheat, dairy and sugars like fructose, lactose and the sweetener, sorbitol. If you've got food intolerances, you'll probably experience abdominal pain, diarrhoea and constipation – all symptoms which fall under the IBS umbrella.

You may also experience depression as fermentation in the gut caused by intolerances can prevent your body from being able to produce tryptothane which produces serotonin (the feel-good hormone that helps keep us happy).

According to Allergy UK, up to 45% of the UK population is affected by food intolerance – the most common being yeast and wheat which are surprisingly present in many products and sauces. The easiest (and free) way to test for intolerances is to remove the suspected food from your diet and see if symptoms improve, then reintroduce it a few weeks later to see if they return (use the trigger diary in chapter 1). It's important to keep an open mind while doing the testing! Always consult your GP if you are planning on drastically altering your diet.

Alternatively, you can pay to have some private food intolerance and allergy tests such as blood tests or kinesiology (a form of energetic testing which checks a person's energetic reaction to certain foods and minerals). Nutritionists may suggest blood tests to check immune reaction (testing blood cells against certain foods which they may react to) and there are several food testing packages on the market.

The York Test food scan is one of the best known. Results are based on the presence and amount of food-specific IgG (immunoglobulin G) antibodies, covering 113 foods analysed by scientists in laboratories (www.yorktest.com). The IgG is a delayed reaction intolerance test – a person may not react to the food in question until several hours or even days later if it shows up in the form of a skin reaction like eczema. This differs from the IgE test which picks up the foods that people have an immediate and dangerous allergic reaction to such as peanuts or shellfish.

You can buy an initial food intolerance test from York Test Laboratories for £9.99. A small pin prick of blood is taken and returned to the labs for analysis. If the test comes back positive (York Test reports that 75% of tests taken are positive), the second step FoodScan 113 test (costing £245 including nutritional advice) can be taken and nutritional advice given.

> 'According to Allergy UK, up to 45% of the UK population is affected by food intolerance – the most common being yeast and wheat which are surprisingly present in many products and sauces.'

Lactose or gluten intolerance

If you suspect you're lactose (sugars found in milk/dairy) or gluten intolerant (around one in 100 people are estimated to have coeliac disease in the UK, a permanent intolerance to gluten, a protein found in wheat, barley and rye), make an appointment to see your GP who can organise the relevant tests. However, note that a positive IgG reaction to gluten is not necessarily diagnostic of coeliac disease.

Menus

Overleaf is a sample IBS-friendly menu compiled by the Head Chef, Klinger Florian at the Viva Mayr resort in Austria. This meal is from their mild clearing diet and is an example of protein food combining. Delicious and healthy, it's ideal for people with IBS or sensitive digestive systems because it's very light. For more information and menus from the Viva Mayr cookery book, see their website at www.viva-mayr.com/en.

Over the next few pages, there are three IBS-friendly breakfast recommendations and a gluten free lunch suggestion from Susie Perry, nutritional therapist.

Filet of organic wild salmon on a bed of fresh spinach and carrot mash with basil oil

(serves 4)

4 filets of organic wild salmon
¼ litre organic vegetable stock
400g fresh organic spinach
200g organic carrots
½ tbsp butter
Pinch of rock salt
Fresh basil
Organic virgin hemp oil (available from a good health food store)
Fresh lemon grass and a pinch of fresh ginger
Fresh nutmeg
Spinach

Slowly heat the organic vegetable stock in a Teflon coated frying pan/wok. Salt salmon filets with rock salt and put into the organic stock. Cover the pan/wok with a lid and simmer for a few minutes. Cook on a low heat.

Fresh spinach and carrot mash

Wash the fresh spinach and remove any hard stalks. Melt the butter in a saucepan and add the spinach for 1-2 minutes until tender. Season and add fresh ground nutmeg. Wash, peel and chop carrots. Cover the carrots with water in a small saucepan, cover with a lid and simmer for 5-7 minutes until tender. Mash or blend in a food processor. Add fresh ginger or lemongrass and season with rock salt. Blend the hemp oil with a small bunch of basil and rock salt until you have green oil. Serve the fish on a bed of spinach and carrot mash, and sprinkle with fresh hemp oil.

Creamy fennel soup with fresh dill

(serves 4)

400g fresh organic fennel
1 litre organic vegetable stock or water
Rock salt
1 small bunch of fresh organic dill

Wash the fennel and chop two thirds of it. Place the rest in a juicer. Boil the stock/water in a saucepan. Add the chopped fennel and boil until tender. Blend in a food processor until very fine and season to taste. Add rock salt and serve with fresh dill.

Millet souffle

(Ideal for wheat/gluten intolerant or vegetarian diets)

150g Millet (or Quinoa)
250g Celeriac (or carrots, courgettes)
2 eggs (just the yolk)
Pinch of rock salt
Sprinkle of nutmeg

Rinse the millet under running water and simmer for 20 minutes (use roughly 2 cups of water to 1 cup of millet). Cook the celeriac/vegetables in water until tender then blend in a food processor. Add the millet, egg yolks, herbs, rock salt and nutmeg. Beat the egg white and fold into the millet mixture. Put the mixture into small soufflé pots on a tray in the oven and bake for 25 minutes at 170oC. Serve with broccoli and leafy greens like spinach and drizzle with olive or fresh hemp oil.

Wheat free bread recipe

1 kg Buckwheat flour (Quinoa or Millet could also be used)
1 tbsp cream of tartar
Approximately 1 litre of water
Pinch of rock salt

Mix the ingredients into a soft pastry and leave for 45 minutes. Mould into small round patties and place on a baking tray. Bake in the oven for 15-18 minutes, at around 175°C.

Peppermint and ginger tea

(for trapped wind and pain)

Handful fresh peppermint
3 slices fresh root ginger

Boil a large mug of hot water and add the peppermint and ginger. Allow to infuse and cool slightly for 10 minutes before drinking.

High fibre porridge

(for constipation)

3 tbsp porridge oats
1 tsp oat bran
3 chopped prunes
1 tsp flax seeds soaked overnight in water
½ chopped pear
300ml milk or milk alternative

Add all the ingredients to a pan and bring to the boil, reduce heat and simmer for 3-4 minutes, adding more liquid if necessary to reach the consistency that you like. This porridge is high in soothing soluble fibre which helps to improve bowel function and regularity.

Settling probiotic smoothie

(for diarrhoea)

3 tbsp natural probiotic yoghurt (cows, sheep, goats or soya yoghurt is fine)
3 slices of fresh pineapple, peeled
2 tsp slippery elm powder
150ml pressed apple juice

Blend all the ingredients together until smooth, adding more apple juice if needed. Probiotic yoghurt contains lactobacillus bacteria which help to boost your friendly gut flora. Pineapple contains enzymes that help boost digestion and slippery elm helps to reduce gut inflammation.

Gluten free quinoa mint salad

(aids digestion and is a good source of protein)

50g Quinoa
2 finely sliced salad onions
2 handfuls of peas
10 king prawns
12 green beans (chopped)
200 ml of chicken stock
2 tsp olive oil

For the dressing
3 tbsp olive oil
2 tbsp chopped mint
1 tbsp white wine vinegar
1 tsp wholegrain mustard
Pinch of salt and pepper

Boil the quinoa with the chicken stock and reduce the heat to simmer for 12-15 minutes or until it is soft and cooked. Drain and set aside to cool. Lightly stir fry the onions, green beans, peas and king prawns in the olive oil then set aside to cool. Mix up the minty dressing and all the cooled ingredients with it before serving.

Summing Up

There's no doubt that what you eat has a huge impact on your digestive health as well as your overall health and wellbeing, however there can be barriers to changing your eating patterns and your diet. Cost is an obvious one, especially at times of economic crisis, but many supermarkets offer special deals on fruit and vegetables to support the 'Five a Day' recommendation, so eating healthily doesn't necessarily have to be expensive!

It can also be challenging to eliminate caffeine, alcohol, fried food or sugar, but with time and determination you can reap the rewards. Other subtle changes can also be made to reduce your IBS symptoms: eating your main meal at lunch time or avoiding eating late at night, making a concerted effort to chew more efficiently and taking the recommended supplements to aid smooth digestion.

One word of warning – if you're eliminating foods, remember to make sure you're still getting a balanced diet and not existing on supplements alone (or on rice and water because you've come to your own conclusion that nearly all foods trigger your IBS!). Consult your GP before making any drastict changes to your diet.

10

IBS in the 21st Century

How busy is your life?

Most of us are always on the go. We're living in a fast-paced, do-it-all, want-it-all kind of culture. Although technology advancements have been phenomenal in the past few decades, are they really making us happier, more balanced people? The things that are supposed to improve our lives and make us feel less stressed seem to just be adding more stress and preventing an effective work/life balance.

The freedom and time to regenerate and relax after a long day's work is essential if we want to feel relaxed, balanced and healthy, but these days we have less and less time to do so. After leaving work for the day, or even when on holiday, you can be on call 24/7 with access to emails from almost anywhere in the world. The result is that we rarely get to truly 'escape' the rat race.

Overload

A certain amount of stress is necessary in life but when we feel too much pressure it can be overwhelming. When the brain becomes overwhelmed by something that happens (or by a negative thought), chemicals are released which act on the nerves in the colon.

These chemicals can cause our intestines to contract or spasm, and the spasms speed up or slow down the digestive system – resulting in diarrhoea or constipation (respectively).

Most people (even those with normal-functioning digestive systems) are affected by anxiety, nerves and stress and need to dash to the toilet several times before making a speech or attending an important interview.

However, if the stress occurs over a long period of time, the brain will go into overload and release too many chemicals. This can lead to excess gas, bloating, cramping and abdominal pain.

Stress and digestion

'You can retrain your eating programme for greater digestive health but you need to be committed to changing your lifestyle too.'

Dr Harald Stossier, medical director of the VIVA centre, The Viva Mayr Health Resort, Austria.

When we're stressed, blood is pulled out of the digestive system as it rushes to the heart and other muscles to prepare the body for dynamic action, like running away from a dinosaur! This is the body going into fight/flight mode.

Therefore, it's really important to eat when you feel calm, relaxed and unhurried – eating when you feel stressed means there's no blood in the stomach to help with digestion and your body can't produce digestive enzymes.

Chapter 9 discussed the importance of chewing food slowly and avoiding drinking with your meal because it can interfere with digestion. Most of us enjoy a glass (or two) of wine with our meals, but alcohol is one of the stimulants to avoid if you want your IBS to improve.

To cut it out completely is an unrealistic goal, so why not aim to take a few small sips during the meal and wait for around 10 to 20 minutes after eating before drinking again? Moderation is the name of the game here.

Anxiety and sleeplessness

The body is a complex machine which needs to regenerate each night. A lack of sleep and sufficient rest will sooner or later have a negative impact on your system.

Sleeping at night is nature's offering for us to be healthy and to live long lives, but many of us today experience disturbed nights because of cares and worries, being woken up in the night or simply because there are not enough hours in the day to fit everything in!

Caffeine, chocolate, sugar and alcohol are some of the worst offenders for disrupting sleep, along with a stressful day and worrying about something you did in the past or are about to do.

Several cups of coffee may well get you going in the mornings but over a continued period of time, insufficient rest and a poor diet will lead to physical and mental exhaustion and could result in other problems.

Break the cycle

In the early hours of the morning your worries are guaranteed to seem far worse. It will be difficult to sleep if your head is full of irrational fears and worries.

Try to cut back on the amount of tea and coffee you drink, especially avoiding caffeine after 2pm, switching to herbal teas and lots of water to stay hydrated. One method which helps with worry during the night is to place a notepad and pen beside your bed and write the thoughts and feelings down when you think of them. You can then deal with them in the morning when you're likely to be feeling more logical and rational, therefore better able to deal with them.

Chill out

There are many things you can try to help you relax and enjoy a better night's sleep. Some gentle exercise before bedtime, meditation or listening to some relaxation CDs can help, as can avoiding watching the news or reading the papers late at night. Instead, read a novel for some escapism or something which inspires you. For more information on getting a good night's sleep, see *Insomnia – The Essential Guide* (Need2Know).

Hypnotherapy is one of the most effective treatments for breaking the cycle of stress, anxiety and insomnia. As well as teaching the mind and body to relax through hypnotic suggestion, it can help you to deal with specific stresses and anxieties by learning new ways of dealing with them on an unconscious level.

These learned patterns of behaviour can then be used by the conscious mind to help you better deal with stressful situations when they occur.

Getting help with depression and anxiety

We all get sad from time to time and it's natural to feel depressed after a traumatic event such as the death of a loved one, exams, losing your job or going through marital or relationship problems.

'Using hypnosis as a tool for relaxation, combined with creating the powerful belief that you can heal yourself, can help to control and reduce the symptoms of IBS.'

Andrew Spence, solution-focused hypnotherapist and life coach, The Spence Practice, East Sussex.

According to the National Association of Counsellors, Hypnotherapists and Psychotherapists (NACHP), many of the side effects or symptoms of stress and depression overlap, resulting in many people concluding that they're depressed (and explaining the vast amount of TCAs being used today).

There are some subtle differences between stress and depression. When you feel stressed you're likely to feel overwhelmed, impatient, frustrated and tired. You'll probably experience mood swings, a lack of sense of humour, headaches, skin problems and feelings of worthlessness or failing. However, if you're suffering with depression you're more likely to feel persistently sad and tired, have trouble concentrating, feel a loss of interest in your daily activities and unable to see anything positive about the future.

Feelings of depression can also be dietary-related. Fermentation in the gut (caused by intolerances) can prevent your body from being able to produce tryptothane which in turn produces serotonin. Serotonin is the feel-good hormone which helps to keep us happy, so it's worth exploring the dietary route to treat your depression.

For more information on depression, see *Depression – The Essential Guide* (Need2Know).

Alternatives to antidepressants

The British Society of Gastroenterology recommends psychological therapies for patients who suffer with stress, anxiety, panic attacks, sleep problems and depression. The great news is that stress management, behavioural therapy and hypnosis have all been proved as extremely effective treatments.

If you're feeling stressed or depressed, ask your GP to refer you to a trained counsellor or recommend some private or low-cost counselling options. The talking therapies can be really effective in replacing negative thoughts and attitudes with more positive ones, in turn reducing stress, anxiety and the inability to sleep. CBT is a particularly effective treatment for the emotional aspects of IBS.

Support from friends and family

If you're feeling tired, fed up and embarrassed by the physical symptoms of IBS, as well as some of the psychological symptoms like anxiety, depression, headaches and exhaustion, the chances are that your friends and family are feeling concerned about you. More often, when you can see others worrying about you it can add to your stress. There's more about coping with relationships and supporting someone with IBS in chapter 12.

Action points

It can take some motivation and effort but look at the list below and consider what you could realistically change today.

How about starting with...

- Making a commitment to eat regular meals, sitting down properly and dedicating at least half an hour to eating. Choosing smaller portions will also put less pressure on your digestive system.

- Ensuring you're comfortable when eating – the last thing you want when you're tucking into your meal is a tight pair of jeans digging into your gut. Change into something comfy and loose. If you're going out for a smart dinner, opt for empire line dresses or tops rather than pinched-in skirts or trousers. If trousers are too tight, undo the top button and cover up with your suit jacket or a loose top!

- Cutting back on caffeine, alcohol and cigarettes. These are stress triggers and we all know it's a myth that they help relax us. Instead, drink lots of water and herbal teas to stay hydrated. However, try to avoid drinking too much before, during or after your meal as this can interfere with efficient digestion, as discussed in chapter 9.

- Becoming familiar with when your IBS symptoms are worse. If you tend to get diarrhoea in the mornings, try to avoid scheduling important interviews, meetings or commitments at that time. If possible, choose familiar places to have the meetings.

- Listening to what your body needs – which therapies or treatments appeal the most and which are within your budget? Once you've made a plan to start feeling better, you're on the way to controlling your IBS rather than letting it control you.

- Listening to and respecting your body's needs and avoiding 'holding it in' or straining when you go to the toilet.

- Learning how to meditate. Search the Internet for courses nearby that can help you learn these skills such as the London Meditation Centre (see help list).

- Practising Savasana (corpse pose, opposite) at bedtime – you may find you've fallen asleep well before you reach the end of the instructions!

'If you're feeling stressed or depressed, ask your GP to refer you to a trained counsellor or recommend some private or low-cost counselling options.'

Get ready for bed and remove the pillow from behind your head so that you're lying completely flat. Place your fingertips on your belly and start to focus on your breathing, feeling it rise up as you inhale and drop down as you exhale. This has a hypnotic effect and will probably make you feel drowsy. If lying on your back isn't comfortable, lie on your front, again remove the pillow, and turn your face to the right or left, with arms at your sides.

After a few breath cycles, start to consciously relax the body from the toes upwards, picturing each part of the body softening and relaxing more and more. In your mind, say to yourself 'my right foot is relaxed', 'my left foot is relaxed', 'my knees are relaxed', 'my thighs are relaxed', 'my hips are relaxed' and so on. Carry on all the way up your body including the lower back, middle back, upper back and shoulders, neck, right arm, right hand/wrist/fingers and left hand/wrist/fingers, the back of the head, forehead, brow, ears, eyes, nose, jaw and face.

Roll your eyes up under the closed lids, let the lower jaw go slack and relax the tongue in the mouth. Every single muscle will begin to relax and your entire body will feel limp and lifeless (hence the name corpse pose!).

After a few moments, turn your attention to relaxing your nervous system, which is much more difficult to relax than the muscles of the body. Try to develop a feeling of letting go. Picture waves of warm relaxation flowing over your body. Imagine that you're sinking into the soft, comforting bed.

Notice your breath, feeling the ebb and flow as you breathe in and out and the sensation of the belly rising and falling back down with each breath.

Now, try to send your mind away from your surroundings, detaching yourself completely from your daily life and responsibilities. Transport yourself to a peaceful and beautiful place (either somewhere you've been on holiday, a picture you've seen or an imaginary place that springs to mind).

Finally, switch off all thoughts or pictures and make your mind blank – just for a few seconds. This can be difficult to do at first but the more you persevere, the easier it becomes to clear the mind and feel deep relaxation of the mind and body.

Yogic relaxation exercise adapted by Sarah Dawson (www.karmiyoga.com).

Summing Up

Whether or not stress is a factor in causing IBS, there's no doubt that the symptoms of IBS can cause us to feel stressed due to the embarrassment and dreaded 'what ifs'. If you've realised that your IBS symptoms are related to a job that you can't stand, a difficult relationship at work, school or home, then it's time to take action – tackling the stress in your life is a good start in helping to reduce your IBS symptoms. There are more tips about coping with the psychological side of IBS in chapters 11 and 12.

You may not be able to control the things in life which make you stressed, so make your goal to change the way that you handle situations so you can feel more relaxed, more of the time.

11

The Brain and IBS

There's a strong relationship between external events and gastrointestinal symptoms. Although it isn't entirely certain that stress causes IBS, one thing for sure is that many of the IBS symptoms cause us to feel stressed due to the embarrassment, anxiety and worry!

Wouldn't it be great to be in control of your nerves and consequently of your IBS symptoms? This is entirely possible through hypnotherapy and mind-over-matter techniques.

However, hypnotherapy isn't a quick-fix magical cure, and your IBS probably won't disappear in one dazzling session! A hypnotherapist can show you the way but ultimately it's up to you to use the training and tools afterwards. If you do, there's every chance of seeing remarkable improvement.

Butterflies

Most of us are familiar with that fluttering feeling of butterflies in our stomach and everyone feels stressed or anxious sometimes – even people with a healthy, functioning digestive system can be affected by nerves before a speech, their wedding day, exams, a date or a job interview.

While our bowels can be irritated by food or drinking contaminated water, it's also strongly recognised that the nervous system can impact the digestive system and trigger the physical (and psychological) symptoms of IBS.

A two-way process

The gut and brain are not separate, disconnected parts of the body. The gastro-intestinal tract (GI tract) contains a network of nerves, and clinical studies have proved that if these nerves experience sensitivity this can trigger changes in the brain that affect our moods. Equally, anxious thoughts in the brain can trigger exaggerated responses in the gut.

Feel-good chemicals

Serotonin is a chemical neurotransmitter that regulates the movement and sensitivity of the gut. It's vital to have the correct amount of this chemical for our bowels to function correctly. Abnormal levels of serotonin can disrupt bowel patterns – if serotonin levels are too high diarrhoea can occur, and if they're too low it's possible to become constipated.

Fight/flight responses

We know that when the brain triggers the fight/flight response in the body the digestive system shuts down. Digesting food uses up lots of energy and the last thing we want is our body trying to process our lunch when we need to be running from danger, sailing through our driving test or performing an awesome best man's speech!

When we're in this stressed state, blood rushes to the heart and other muscles to prepare the body for action. This is fine every now and again but over a prolonged period of time it can be very damaging to the body.

If there's a lack of blood in the stomach, your body can't produce digestive enzymes and you won't be able to absorb all the necessary nutrients and vitamins you need to function optimally. The resulting digestive problems can trigger any of the IBS symptoms.

'During hypnotherapy the mind becomes relaxed and stressful situations become more manageable. As a result, the immune and digestive systems begin to function more effectively.'

Cat Murphy, hypnotherapist, Brighton.

Why hypnotherapy is so effective for IBS

In 2005, a study conducted by Peter Whorwell, a professor of medicine and gastroenterology at the University of Manchester, found that gut-directed hypnosis was an extremely effective treatment for IBS patients.

Two hundred and fifty patients (all of whom had suffered from IBS for more than two years) received 12 one-hour hypnotherapy sessions and also sessions about what causes IBS and how the digestive system works. For 70% of patients, hypnotherapy was an effective treatment for IBS.

However, until hypnotherapy for IBS is widely available on the NHS, you'll need to find a private hypnotherapist. Check with your GP, ask around for recommendations or contact the National Society of Counsellors, Hypnotherapists and Psychotherapists for some advice (www.nachp.org). You could also check with the General Hypnotherapy Standards Council (www.ghsc.co.uk), the British Institute of Hypnotherapy and NLP (www.users.globalnet.co.uk/~bih) or the NHS Directory of Complementary and Alternative Practitioners (www.nhsdirectory.org).

How it works

The hypnotic state is one of deep relaxation where stress is reduced and every organ, function and system of the body slows down. During the hypnotherapy session patients learn to influence the gut function and gain understanding of how the brain regulates gut activity. This enables them to take control of the IBS symptoms, rather than having the IBS symptoms control them.

Andrew Spence, Dip PDMSM, MNCH (Acc) of the Spence Practice, East Sussex (www.thespencepractice.co.uk) is a solution-focused hypnotherapist and life coach. Approximately 75% of his patients suffer from anxiety/stress-related conditions, including IBS. Following is a description of what is likely to happen in one of his hypnotherapy consultations.

'I provide a free initial consultation in order to assess whether hypnotherapy would be appropriate. This assessment includes a detailed case history, presenting symptoms, establishing whether or not IBS has been diagnosed by the medical profession, finding out what tests have been taken to rule out other digestive conditions and details of any medication being taken.

'By learning tools which enable you to relax deeply, you can start to regain control over your thoughts, feelings and emotions and send the correct signals from your nervous system to the digestive system.'

Andrew Spence of the Spence Practice, East Sussex, a solution-focused hypnotherapist and life coach.

'It's important to ascertain personality traits, thinking styles, behaviour patterns and emotional resilience. It can also be helpful to know what was happening in the patient's life before symptoms first appeared. Lifestyle issues such as diet, sleep and ability to cope with stress are also factors taken into consideration.

'I take a holistic approach and explain the connection between mind and body, and how the nervous system can and does impact on the digestive system through the body's 'fight or flight' response (in other words how the nervous system responds to the stress alarm and causes the digestive system to malfunction).

'I help my clients to understand how the digestive system functions and how learning new coping strategies for dealing with stress results in a calmer, more relaxed person. I explain that it is important to realise that we can and do control the digestive system subconsciously.

'Hypnosis is a highly effective tool for managing the symptoms of IBS. Hypnosis is a state of inner absorption, like meditation or a controlled daydream state. It is natural and safe – we sometimes experience this daydream state while carrying out day-to-day activities like driving a car while on autopilot.

'During this heightened state of inner awareness we are more susceptible to be influenced by positive suggestions and to using our creativity to solve problems. Hypnosis can be used to help a patient speed up or slow down the digestive system, depending on whether the main symptom is diarrhoea or constipation.

'Hypnotherapy can be effectively combined with other techniques such as cognitive behaviour therapy (CBT) to help change thoughts and beliefs. I could combine it with the emotional freedom technique (EFT) if I am working with an emotional person.

'The treatment is individually tailored to each client. It usually takes between four and eight sessions to achieve a significant improvement in the severity and frequency of symptoms. I focus on relieving stress, teaching self-hypnosis and visualisation techniques such as visualising the gut working harmoniously, using metaphors like a gently flowing river or a well-lubricated car engine. Some of the hypnotherapy sessions are recorded onto CD for patients to listen to at home on a daily basis.'

(Consultation charges vary dependent on location. Expect to pay from £50 upwards.)

Autogenic therapy

Autogenic therapy (AT) was developed in the 20th century by a psychiatrist and neurologist called Dr Schultz. AT involves learning some simple mental exercises which turn off the 'fight or flight' mechanism in the body and bring about a deeply relaxed state of being in a similar way that yoga or meditation can. AT is similar to meditation (and hypnosis) because it involves a change in consciousness – however, there are no spiritual or religious goals – the purpose is simply to feel relaxed!

As a result, AT is a holistic and complementary approach to treating IBS and a range of psychosomatic and psychological issues, reducing the effects of stress by inducing deep relaxation and retraining the mind to calm itself. The great thing about it is that once you've learnt how to do it you can induce a deep state of relaxation at will. According to the British Autogenic Society (www.autogenic-therapy.org.uk), AT is one of the most scientifically proven complementary therapies, yet one of the least known, and perhaps a good alternative if you're put off by the spiritual or religious aspects associated with meditation or yoga.

Summing Up

Most of us lead busy lives and stress is never very far behind. The value of taking the time to learn some new tools and techniques which will help calm your mind and physically relax your body cannot be underestimated. You can help reduce your stress levels by practising the AT technique, learning to meditate, practising yoga or visiting a hypnotherapist. All of these are empowering treatment options which can help reduce any of the IBS symptoms. You'll need to practise regularly and utilise the tools, preferably on a day-to-day basis, to really see the benefits.

12

Coping and Living with IBS

Depending on the severity of your symptoms, IBS can have a negative impact on the quality of your life. In addition to the embarrassing and inconvenient physical symptoms, the psychological symptoms like anxiety, headaches and trouble sleeping can seriously wear you down.

Socialising

For many people, IBS symptoms are so severe that they dare not leave the house for fear of having an 'incident'. This could mean the mere suggestion of joining friends for social get-togethers where everyone else can happily tuck into spicy Indian or Thai cuisine and drink beer or wine with abandonment is at best difficult, and at worst out of the question.

However, the more you worry about having diarrhoea or abdominal pain when you're in social situations, the less you'll want to go out. It's a vicious circle because the more you worry, the more your IBS symptoms are likely to worsen.

Preparation

If there's a big event, dinner or party coming up which you really want to go to, prepare for it. Aim to be as relaxed as possible beforehand, make sure you get plenty of exercise, eat the right kind of foods (ones that won't trigger bad symptoms), try some of the meditation, breathing and visualisation techniques at the end of this chapter and go to bed early so that you're well rested.

Without being paranoid, find out where the toilets are in the restaurant/café/bar. Order wisely, remembering which foods and drinks could trigger symptoms. If you fancy a glass of wine, don't deny yourself too rigidly but learn to know when to avoid the things that could bring on a bout.

'The only way to get rid of the fear of doing something is to go out and do it.'
Susan Jeffers, author.

Quit the 'what ifs'

Start trying to focus on the expectation of things going well, rather than on the 'What if I can't find a toilet or have an accident, get excruciating pain and need to lie down?' which can trap you in a vicious cycle and prevent you from leading a balanced and enjoyable life.

Anxiety is caused by looking ahead and thinking of the worst possible outcome, but if you turn it around and learn to create positive anticipation, i.e. things going well and your digestive system functioning better, then this is much more likely to be the case.

Feel the fear and do it anyway

As Susan Jeffers says in her book *Feel the Fear and Do It Anyway* (Rider & Co), confronting your fears is better than feeling paralysed, stuck and held back from living your life.

So why not start 'trusting' your digestive system and visualising it functioning healthily and smoothly? Ask yourself 'what's the worst thing that can happen?' then positively affirm that whatever happens, you'll handle it.

Learn some of the tools to cope with anxiety – see the visualisation, muscle relaxation and breathing exercises at the end of this chapter. However, if it makes you feel more in control, take some back-up items like Imodium, tissues/wet wipes, peppermint or chamomile teabags or anti-spasmodics in case of abdominal pain.

Not suffering alone

Knowing that you're not alone with your IBS is a great comfort, so checking out the many different online forums for IBS sufferers could be useful to help you overcome isolation. See if there is an IBS support group in your area for sharing experiences with other people in the same situation. If there isn't one nearby, why not set one up yourself?

There's a list of IBS charities and organisations at the back of the book in the help list. While it's good to share stories with other people, it's also important to keep your interest in IBS balanced, focusing on how to conquer it and live life fully.

Travelling

Your IBS symptoms could be (or in the past have been) so severe and frequent that your whole life seems to revolve around your digestive system and making sure you've got access to decent toilets.

Hopefully now you'll be able to see that there is light at the end of the tunnel and you can learn how to control the physical and psychological aspects of IBS through mind-over-matter and hypnosis techniques. Both of which can easily be learnt and practised at home, while on a train or waiting in a queue.

The breathing and visualisation techniques can help overcome the anxiety and stress related to long bus, plane, train or car journeys and can help restore confidence in taking holidays and flights again.

Of course, these techniques can't take away the risk of getting sick while abroad and, unfortunately, some people's IBS symptoms seem to start after a holiday or where they caught viral or bacterial gastroenteritis.

Most infections caught abroad are contracted via food, passed on via the people handling the food or by unclean water. Take some precautions: drink only bottled mineral water if tap water is unfit for drinking, avoid ice cubes and remember to clean your teeth with bottled water too.

It's advisable to avoid really spicy dishes, unpeeled fruit or vegetables and to stay well hydrated in hot countries. As a back-up you could ask your GP to prescribe you some antibiotics like ciprofloxacin (ciproxin) – if they're taken as soon as diarrhoea begins, they can seriously reduce the severity and length of a gut infection.

Managing at home

If you've decided it's necessary to address your diet to relieve IBS symptoms, the support of your partner, family and friends is essential as it will mean an alteration in eating habits and perhaps more time and effort to prepare.

If, for example, you discover that wheat exacerbates your symptoms, this will invariably mean a total overhaul of what you normally eat for breakfast, lunch and dinner which in this country tend to be based around wheat cereals, toast, sandwiches and pasta. You can still have special types of bread and cereals but substitutes will need to be made.

Shop around until you find the alternative wheat-free bread or pasta that you prefer. Look on the Internet for websites offering wheat/lactose/sugar/gluten free menus and check out the many 'free-from' cookery books in your library or online at websites like Amazon.

The changes can be hard, especially if the rest of the family are tucking into crusty white toast and the smell of croissants drives you mad! It will take a lot of willpower and commitment to stick to your new diet – this is where you should draw on the support of a friend or your nutritional therapist.

'If you've decided it's necessary to address your diet to relieve IBS symptoms, the support of your partner, family and friends is essential as it will mean an alteration in eating habits and perhaps more time and effort to prepare.'

Managing at work, school or college

If meetings and appointments cause a bout of diarrhoea or abdominal pain, it can be really challenging to maintain a professional persona and, not least, a normal working routine. If severe diarrhoea, constipation or pain is affecting you on a regular basis, you may often be missing from your desk which is particularly stressful if you have to explain yourself to an unsympathetic boss or teacher.

You may feel worried about going to school or sitting in lectures or meetings where it isn't easy or convenient to just slip out and go to the toilet. Speaking to your boss or teacher and explaining what is happening is better than just disappearing without an explanation.

You might also want to make an appointment to speak to your boss or someone in the Human Resources department to explain your situation and to see what could be done to help make things more 'workable', for example working from home or coming in later in the morning if symptoms are particularly bad first thing. Meanwhile, build in a daily programme of exercise, breathing, visualisation and muscle relaxation to help you gain more control of your symptoms.

Relationships

IBS is a stressful condition and where there's stress there are usually arguments and disagreements – even in the strongest of relationships. But being in a relationship with someone who has IBS can also be difficult. You can make it easier by calmly explaining your understanding of the condition to them and how it affects you.

Hypnotherapist Andrew Spence recommends explaining to your partner, friends and family that your nervous system is impacting on your digestive system more severely than it does for most people.

While it's good to get empathy from friends, family and partners, a balance should be made. Talking about your IBS a lot and using it as an excuse for not doing things gives it the wrong sort of energy. What you want to be doing is directing your energy into treating it and living your life as fully as possible.

Supporting someone with IBS

The best support you can give to someone with IBS is empathy and patience, never invalidating, teasing, hurrying or making a big deal about it if they need to go to the toilet more regularly than you, even if they take ages when they do. Allow them space, time, privacy and the respect they deserve.

Try to be flexible and understanding and suggest meals in restaurants which would have a varied menu, rather than inviting them to spicy Indian or Mexican restaurants which could be embarrassing for them to say no to.

Helping children or teenagers with IBS

Children and teenagers can get constipated if they are exposed to stress at school or home or if they're too busy playing or hanging out with friends that they simply forget to 'go'.

Since insoluble fibre can make bloating, constipation and gas worse, rather than plying your family with more bran and roughage, encourage them to eat more soluble fibre like carrots, spinach, chickpeas, butter beans and grains like quinoa or buckwheat to help the bowels function well.

It is very important for children (and everyone) to drink plenty of water (six to eight cups of water every day) as dehydration can cause constipation. Make sure your child is also drinking plenty of water after a cold or flu as the body will need extra fluids.

'Everyone is affected by anxiety or stress and we all get upset tummies at some point in our lives. You could describe IBS as an extension of a natural bodily reaction irritated by certain food, drinks or stress.'

Andrew Spence of the Spence Practice, East Sussex, a solution-focused hypnotherapist and life coach.

If your child puts off going to the toilet, his/her stools will become dry and uncomfortable, making them want to avoid 'going' even more! However, ignoring the body's needs can upset the system, so it's important to educate your child on the importance of regular trips to the toilet.

Once they get to teenage years, your children probably won't want to hear lectures or discuss going to the bathroom with you. Just try to make sure that they know the basics: it's important to get a good night's rest and that late nights, alcohol, junk food, eating in a hurry and not allowing food to digest before meeting friends to run about or play football can cause problems. You'll have to lead by example here!

'Children and teenagers can get constipated if they are exposed to stress at school or home or if they're too busy playing or hanging out with friends that they simply forget to "go".'

Help at school

It's important to develop a relationship with your child's teacher/tutor and to keep them informed of what your son or daughter is experiencing. Request a 'pass' to enable them to go freely to the toilet to avoid as much embarrassment as possible. This will be easier at primary level when they will just have one teacher in charge of them. If your child is in secondary school, you may need to see the headteacher.

The Gut Trust's website (the national charity for IBS in the UK) has a wealth of helpful tips and advice for parents, children and teenagers, including a junior network support group which was set up by a young boy called Ewan Povell who has suffered with IBS since the age of 11. See their guide to coping at school (a helpful guide for parents) which includes a chart showing what an 'ideal' stool should look like, bringing some humour into a tricky subject. There's also a section with lots of jokes to help keep children amused and positive about overcoming their condition. The website is www. theguttrust.org.

Action points

The following tools can be easily learned and take just a few minutes to practise. You can do them at home or even on a bus or train.

For best results, practice the relaxation/visualisation exercises daily. If your tummy is already squirming about the thought of a special event or presentation, now is the perfect time!

Calming breath exercise

Sitting in a comfortable chair (or lying down) with your feet flat on the ground and your arms by your sides, breathe in through your nose as you count to three in your mind, pause for a moment, then breathe out of the nose to a count of six. Repeat for six breath cycles. This exercise can be done almost anywhere, whenever you feel yourself getting stressed or anxious.

Auto suggestion (muscle relaxation exercise)

This exercise is meant to help the body feel deep relaxation. Firstly, you exaggerate tension in the various muscles of the body before letting go, so that you can feel the contrast of holding tension and then of letting go.

Sitting or lying down, inhale through the nose. As you inhale, raise the right leg a few centimetres from the ground, hold the tension in the leg, flex the foot then point the foot. As you breathe out, drop your leg down heavily, with a sense of 'letting go'.

Do the same with the left leg, then the right arm and the left arm (making a fist with the hands to exaggerate muscle tension), lifting up on the in-breath then exhaling and letting them drop down. Next, inhale and push up your hips, clenching the buttocks, exhaling to relax them. Do the same with the chest, feeling the tension in your shoulders, exhaling to relax them.

Inhale and try to reach your ears with your shoulders, exaggerating the tension, then exhale and relax. Finally, stick your tongue out as far as it will go and make a roaring sound (best done at home, rather than in a public place!). Scan the body from top to toe, sending relaxation instructions to each part, starting with the right and left foot then the legs, pelvis, back, shoulders, arms, hands, neck, head and face.

Visualisation

Find a really inspiring and relaxing picture to use as an 'anchor' – a calming scene to visualise when you feel stressed. It could be a holiday photograph or a country that you'd like to visit. Sitting in a comfortable seat or lying down at home, picture the scene. Imagine you are there and are experiencing the sights and sounds of that place, such as the birds, the smell of flowers or freshly mown grass. After five to 10 minutes, gently open your eyes and move slowly and gently before continuing with your activities.

Summing Up

You're now armed with a range of methods for managing your IBS, whether you're planning a holiday abroad, aiming to improve things at work or school, overhauling your diet or starting to enjoy a social life once more. Preparation, nurturing a positive mental attitude and gaining support from friends, family members or support groups will all contribute to better management of your IBS.

Try to take small steps, acknowledging each success and accepting that some days you may need to cancel social events or travel arrangements. It's better to be realistic than to expect to achieve full control of your IBS all of the time, only to feel frustrated when an unexpected bout of symptoms arrive and stop you in your tracks.

13

Conclusion

B y now you should have a good understanding of IBS and plenty of options for treating it.

Normally this would be the part of the book to quote the latest findings and research projects for an IBS cure. But as you know that IBS is a series of symptoms caused by a functional disorder in the bowels rather than a disease, there isn't actually a cure.

The understanding and treatment of the condition has come a long way in recent years and it's now believed to be entirely possible to reverse IBS.

The best way to do this is to experiment and find out what works best for you on a dietary, lifestyle management and treatment basis.

Word from the experts

The National Institute for Health and Clinical Excellence (NICE) currently recommends anti-spasmodic agents and soluble fibre as the first-line treatments for IBS.

Recent Canadian research (2008) found that peppermint oil was more effective for treating IBS than anti-spasmodics. Lead researcher Dr Alex Ford, from the gastroenterology division at McMaster University in Ontario, recommended two capsules of peppermint oil taken three times each day as a first-line treatment, moving on to anti-spasmodics and fibre if the peppermint oil isn't effective.

Scientific evidence for food elimination diets

In 2004 the journal *Gut* published details about a clinical trial in which patients suffering from IBS followed an exclusion diet after taking the York Test's FoodScan 113 test. The article concluded that a clinically significant result can be achieved by following a food elimination diet based on the levels of IgG reactivity after taking the FoodScan 113 test. Good news if you're planning a dietary overhaul!

Taking a holistic approach

Because IBS can be caused or made worse by external factors, it's important to take into account the psychological and social factors rather than just treating the physical symptoms, remembering that what works for one person doesn't necessarily work for another.

Doctors and health professionals recognise the uniqueness of the condition and are now much more open to recognising the many different treatment options, including the benefits of complementary therapies like acupuncture or gut-directed hypnotherapy.

What's more, due to the revolution of the Internet, we no longer have to rely solely on a flying visit to the doctor's surgery for information about treating the condition. Most of us today can gain instant access to knowledge and research online. That said, it's important not to get too carried away with self-diagnosis or self-prescribing! It's vital to seek professional guidance and advice.

'Doctors and health professionals recognise the uniqueness of the condition and are now much more open to recognising the many different treatment options, including the benefits of complementary therapies like acupuncture or hypnotherapy.'

Reassurance

A big part of treating IBS is being reassured that the symptoms don't indicate a much more serious condition, a point highlighted in chapter 7 by consultant gastroenterologist Dr Suneil Kapadia at New Cross Hospital, Royal Wolverhampton NHS Trust.

Mercury dental fillings

The controversy about mercury fillings being bad for our health flits in and out of the media. Is it possible that they may be causing gastrointestinal problems like IBS?

Mercury is known to be poisonous and for some years there have been concerns about the mercury content of traditional fillings being absorbed into the body. Research has been inconclusive as the percentage of mercury components contained within the silver, amalgam fillings deemed too low to be of any concern.

However, the European Union (EU) recognises that mercury is a danger to people and a directive due to come into effect in 2011 bans the further use of mercury in a variety of products, including dental fillings.

So if you've tried other treatments and not had much success and you've also got a mouthful of mercury and can afford to have the private dental treatment (or you've got dental cover), it may be worth raising the issue with you GP and dentist. They should be able to explain more about the effects of mercury fillings and the pros and cons of having them replaced.

Summing Up

Whatever treatment option you decide to take, whether you go down the psychological route via the talking therapies or via the food elimination and nutritional route (or indeed, both!), you may gain full control over your symptoms and be able to completely forget about IBS.

But – and it's a big but – if your symptoms do come back, try not to feel too disappointed or that you've wasted your time and money. IBS can come and go and if you get fixated on it coming back, the stress and associated negative emotions won't help matters!

For most people, the condition tends to persist long term, with the severity of symptoms changing. If and when your IBS symptoms reappear, go back to the drawing board, look at your diet, your lifestyle and your stress levels and consider whether the same things have triggered it again or if it could be something entirely different.

The bowels are intrinsically linked to the brain, so if your IBS was caused by a particularly stressful experience in the past, it's quite likely that symptoms could reappear in the future if you go through another difficult period. However, if the approach you adopted worked before, do it again!

14

Frequently Asked Questions

How do I know if I've got IBS?

It's vital that you don't self-diagnose. Make an appointment to talk through your symptoms and concerns with your GP and get a proper medical diagnosis.

Can I cure my IBS?

There isn't a cure for IBS as it is a series of symptoms caused by a functional disorder in the bowels, rather than a disease. However, there is a whole range of treatments, medication, approaches and therapies to treat the symptoms of IBS, and health professionals believe it's entirely possible to lessen, ease and even reverse the symptoms.

I have abdominal pain and constipation but they only occur during my period – do I have IBS?

It is possible that you've got IBS. However, if your symptoms are only occurring during your period it's advisable that you see your GP. They may recommend seeing a gynaecologist to rule out any issues in that area before looking at other ways to treat your symptoms.

Why have I got IBS?

'It's vital that you don't self-diagnose. Make an appointment to talk through your symptoms and concerns with your GP and get a proper medical diagnosis.'

No one really knows the exact answer to this question. IBS is believed to be triggered by a number of factors including stress, diet, an imbalance in the gut's flora (due to a course of antibiotics or a parasitic infection) and emotional trauma, as well as a person's attitude to life and ability to manage stress.

How do I find out if I'm intolerant to certain foods?

If you suspect you're lactose (sugars found in milk/dairy) or gluten intolerant (a permanent intolerance to gluten, a protein found in wheat, barley and rye known as coeliac disease), go and see your GP for a blood test. Your GP can also do a food allergy skin prick test to discover immediate allergic reactions to foods like shellfish or nuts. Other intolerance tests can be done privately via a nutritional therapist or via a food testing company like York Test Laboratories.

Do I have to choose between conventional medicine and complementary medicine to treat my IBS?

No, treatments work very well together. However, you should advise your GP/therapist about what you're doing. Nutritional therapist Susie Perry believes that acupuncture, for example, is very effective with nutritional advice if there are emotional issues contributing to the digestive problems and you don't feel like going down the therapist/counsellor route. Acupuncture can reset the adrenal (stress) glands and help settle the mind (and heart) to aid relaxation.

Can IBS lead to other conditions and shorten my life expectancy?

One of the biggest fears for people experiencing IBS symptoms is that there's something more sinister going on or that it could lead to something more serious. According to the Gut Trust (the UK's national IBS charity), IBS isn't going to kill you, nor is it going to increase your likelihood of developing bowel cancer or other bowel conditions. However, since IBS tends to worsen when a person is stressed, if the stress isn't addressed then other problems could potentially occur. If you eat lots of fatty or junk foods, this could lead to heart or other health problems. Health experts say that IBS itself will not lead to anything more serious or harmful.

15

Case Studies

Sarah Dawson – the author

'My IBS symptoms first started at 19 when I left home to study in another city. I believe it was triggered by a combination of factors: a change in diet, the psychological impact of leaving home and missing friends and family and a new routine – as well as a hectic social life which usually involved drinking and late night partying!

'I started to get really bad abdominal pains, gas and bloating. I would be out with friends and be doubled over in pain so would frequently need to go home early and lie down with a hot water bottle until the pain subsided.

'When I went to see my GP, he recommended I eat a bowl of bran cereal each day. I tried this and my belly turned into a balloon! I visited my GP several more times and he suggested anti-spasmodics and some relaxation tapes to help reduce stress and anxiety.

'The tapes were very effective and inspired my interest in the power of the mind as a tool to heal, and also in yoga and meditation. Over the subsequent years, the IBS came and went, usually heightened by events such as exams or relationships.

'I regularly attended yoga classes, swam twice a week throughout my 20s, ate reasonably healthily and occasionally used anti-spasmodics or peppermint oil if a bad bout of stress caused abdominal pains.

'Despite my GP's advice to eat more fibre, brown rice, pasta and bread, it tended to make my symptoms worse. Instead, I ate white bread/pasta/rice and got my fibre from fruit and vegetables.

'At times my IBS completely disappeared, usually when I felt relaxed and happy. However, the symptoms always seemed to return whenever I felt stressed. I often wondered if I was wheat intolerant and would occasionally try eliminating wheat or dairy from my diet for a few weeks to see if anything changed.

'It wasn't until a few years ago while on a press trip to the Viva Mayr health resort in Austria that I discovered my IBS might be due to fructose intolerance (the sugars found in fruit). I ate tons of fruit to compensate for not eating wholemeal bread and brown rice or pasta and I loved honey, pouring it onto yogurt and fruit every morning for breakfast.

'Some people can digest fructose better than others, but if you're sensitive to it, it can remain in the large intestine and ferment. Using applied kinesiology and a breath test to establish whether my breath contained hydrogen and methane, Dr Stossier, the Viva Mayr's medical director, revealed that fructose intolerance was causing fermentation in my colon, resulting in gas, constipation, abdominal pain and bloating symptoms. Other nutrients and vitamins weren't being absorbed properly which explained why I often felt sluggish and a bit depressed.

'I followed the Mayr inner cleansing programme which included learning to eat slowly, chew more efficiently and involved therapies like reflexology to help stimulate my digestive system. I then eliminated fruits for six months, including honey and any dressing or sweetener which included fructose such as maple syrup.

'I increased my intake of vegetables to ensure I was getting enough vitamins and minerals, and very quickly felt a dramatic and positive improvement in my digestive system. After six months I reintroduced some low fructose fruits into my diet such as blueberries, avoiding heavy fructose-rich ones like bananas, apples and pears as these would trigger my symptoms immediately.

'I believe it's been a combination of eating the right foods, avoiding the ones which trigger symptoms, managing stress through regular yoga practice and the occasional massage or reflexology session that has resulted in my control of the IBS. I now rarely experience abdominal pain or any other IBS symptoms.'

Michael*

aged nine from Sussex, as told by his mother Susan* (*names changed for confidentiality)

'Michael has experienced pain in the same place in his stomach ever since he was born which at first we thought was very bad colic. When he was old enough to say a few words, he started to talk of this pain in his tummy and as he got older GPs treated it as reflux, but the medicine made no difference.

'From seven months Michael chose to only accept a controlled diet, eating only a narrow range of food items. He gets very easily aroused (less so now that he is maturing) and feels panicky if he feels a situation is unfair or about to go wrong. Michael gets very ill when he's triggered into one of these anxious states and the undiagnosed pain in the stomach has resulted in many trips to the hospital.

'His stomach pain can come on at any time. When the pain level is intense, it's as though he's having waves of contractions as tears run down his face. As a parent it's extremely hard to see him like this. Sometimes it can last on and off for weeks, even months. He misses up to 15% of school every year and he's sometimes ill during the holidays and weekends.

'It's taken years of going back and forth to various doctors and specialists to try and determine the cause of the pain. However, Michael was recently diagnosed with abdominal migraine, which falls within the IBS spectrum. Although he takes a range of anti-spasmodic medicines, they only dull his pain.

'The GP, gastroenterologist and the mental health consultant have agreed that the best way forward is to help Michael control his anxiety in order to help control the stomach pain. It has been recognised that it's the anxiety which triggers Michael's IBS episodes.

'Michael now attends a child mental health service for cognitive behaviour therapy (CBT) and this is having a really positive impact on all of his symptoms.

'Some time ago, one of the hospitals assessed Michael's anxiety as being brought on by his early life experiences of sudden episodes of ill health which were life threatening, painful, intrusive, frightening and confusing for a baby.

'It has been really beneficial for Michael to be able to talk about his pain and anxiety symptoms and for someone to really listen to him. The biggest and most dramatic change was when the therapist asked Michael to draw what it feels like when he's in pain and to name his fear. This really helped bring the anxiety out into the open and reassure him.

'He's now acquiring tools to manage his anxiety. The emotional freedom technique is great for managing his fear, anxiety and other negative feelings and he now has good self-awareness regarding his symptoms and what's going on.

'All in all, things are definitely improving, especially with his ability to manage his emotions. I have started a counselling course to better understand how we can support him as a family. After nine long years we're finally seeing light at the end of the tunnel for Michael and his anxiety-related IBS.'

Help List

IBS charities, health associations and dietary advice

British Association for Applied Nutrition and Nutritional Therapy (BANT)
27 Old Gloucester Street, London, WC1N 3XX
Tel: 08706 061284
www.bant.org.uk
The professional association for nutritional therapists. Their website provides information for the public and lists practitioners.

British Dietetic Association (BDA)
5th Floor, Charles House, 148/9 Great Charles Street Queensway, Birmingham, B3 3HT
Tel: 0121 200 8080
www.bda.uk.com
The BDA is a professional association for dieticians. Their website has lots of vital food facts and is a great resource for learning how to eat a balanced diet for optimum health. It's packed with information on medical conditions, allergies, the truth about alcohol and how the food we eat can affect our moods.

British Nutrition Foundation (BNF)
High Holborn House, 52–54 High Holborn, London, WC1V 6RQ
Tel: 020 7557 7930
www.nutrition.org.uk
The BNF is a registered charity which promotes health and wellbeing through the science of nutrition and physical exercise. Their website is a great resource for the general public and schools with up-to-date dietary and nutritional news, facts, figures, recipes and information about leading a healthy lifestyle.

British Society of Gastroenterology (BSG)
3 St Andrews Place, Regent's Park, London, NW1 4LB
Tel: 020 7935 3150
www.bsg.org.uk
The BSG helps to promote high standards of patient care in gastroenterology. Their website has clinical information on digestive disorders and research.

CORE

3 St Andrews Place, London, NW1 4LB

Tel: 020 7486 0341

www.gutscharity.org.uk

This is the only UK charity that funds research into gut, liver, intestinal and bowel illnesses. It aims to provide the public with clear facts and information about these conditions. See their website for case studies, research and information about fundraising events.

The IBS Network

Unit 1, 16 SOAR Works, 14 Knutton Road, Sheffield, S5 9NU

Tel: 0114 272 3253

We are the national charity supporting people living with Irritable Bowel Syndrome. Our mission is to provide information and advice, working alongside healthcare professionals to facilitate self-management. Thanks to your donations, we help thousands of IBS sufferers to live well with this debilitating condition.

The Natural Health Advisory Service

PO Box 117, Rottingdean, East Sussex, BN51 9BG

Tel: 01273 609699

www.naturalhealthas.com

Another very useful resource for IBS and PMS formerly known as the Women's Nutritional Advisory Service. See the website for information about conquering IBS and PMS through a healthy diet and complementary therapies.

Patrick Holford

Carters Yard, Wandsworth High Street, London, SW18 4JR

www.patrickholford.com

Leading nutritionist's website packed with information and advice about healthy eating.

Susie Perry

Tel: 01825 724151

info@nurturingspirit.co.uk

www.nurturingspirit.co.uk

Nurturing Spirit is a nutritional therapy company based in East Sussex.

Susie's website provides information about treating IBS and other digestive conditions through nutrition and testing for intolerances.

Viva Mayr

Centre for Modern Mayr Medicine, Seepromenade 11, A-9082 Maria Worth, Carinthia, Austria
Tel: +43 4273 31117
office@viva-mayr.com
www.viva-mayr.com/en
The website explains more about the Mayr approach to optimum digestion.